BUNNETICS

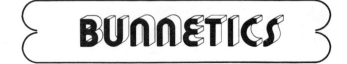

How To Shape Your Buns

Cal del Pozo

A DOLPHIN BOOK
Doubleday & Company, Inc., Garden City, New York
1982

*Cal del Pozo's clothes supplied by The Crow's Nest, New York City.
Darlene La Preste's clothes supplied by Capezio Ballet Makers, Inc.*

*Drawings by William Ronalds
Photographs by George Bennett*

ISBN: 0-385-17974-X
Library of Congress Catalog Card Number 81–43580
Copyright © 1982 by Cal del Pozo

To my parents, for the life they gave me; to the Clark A. Weaver family and the city of Perrysburg, Ohio, for saving it; and to Kathryn, for her enduring love.

I would like to thank the following people for their cooperation and assistance: Tim Pearson, Gary Pool, Susan Schader, Eugene Stavis, Sally Gouverneur, David Bober, Dr. Michael Weinstein, Dr. Paul Scoles, John Caranci, and a special thanks to my editor, Nan Grubbs, without whose support and encouragement a lot of buns would have stayed closeted. Thanks also to all my students whose buns have suffered the experimentations of their Bunophobic teacher.

Contents

Introduction

My name is Cal del Pozo and I am a dancer who suffers from Bunophobia: the fear of fat and sagging buns. As a cure I have taken on the task of making ugly buns beautiful, and I spend a great deal of time doing so through the use of a method I have named Bunnetics. Its purpose is to keep all the buns in the world in shape and thus eradicate the dreadful disease from which I suffer.

The Bunnetics program is simple to follow, but before I tell you more about it there are a few personal questions I must ask you. How are your buns? Are they drooping a little bit? Are you satisfied with the looks they get? Have you even taken a good look at them lately? Come on, place your hand over them and press a little. Sort of soft, eh? Do you remember when (or if) they were a little harder? Well, don't let it trouble you. Soon they are going to be in better shape than you ever dreamed. This book you are holding has the answer to correcting years of neglect.

But first try this:

The Shifter

Sit down, if you're not sitting already. Shift your weight over to the left leg. Do it slowly—I promise you that no one will notice. Now tighten your left cheek real hard. You must do it for 10 counts. Now, go! 1-2-3-4-5-6-7-8-9-10. Relax for 5 counts and do it again. Felt real good didn't it? And it went unnoticed, except, that is, by your right cheek. So give it a little loving too. Shift your weight to the right and repeat the whole thing. You see, buns are muscles, and as such need work to stay strong and firm.

The Shifter is just one of the Pre-Bun conditioning exercises you will find scattered throughout the first part of the book. Do each Pre-Bun exercise as you come across it, so that as you read your buns are getting ready for the exercises in Buns One.

Here is another, ready?

The Clincher

Stand with your feet parallel, about a foot apart, and flex your knees just a little. Now tuck your lower abdomen in and hold tight, then squeeze your buns together, and now tighten your thighs. Hold for 1-2-3-4-5. Relax. One more time. Go! Two of those an hour and in a week's time the results will amaze you.

How about one for the road?

The Bun Dimpler

Sit again, and press your legs together, squeezing your buns at the same time. Press and squeeze for 2 counts then relax for 1 count. Do it 10 times. See? You are smiling. Buns have a direct line to the mouth. When they feel loved, you smile, and when they are neglected, they just pull you right down to that chair and get bigger and bigger.

If you are in fairly good shape, Bunnetics will help you stay fit with just a few minutes a day. If you are like most people and leave nice buns and a slender body to the imagination, this is your chance to let your mind turn fantasy into reality. As you read on you will find that Bunnetics is closely related to the creation of pictures in your mind. Throughout the following chapters you will find out a lot about those two gorgeous creatures that give us a lot of support even though we constantly leave them behind. The time is now.

My buns thank you, and in a little time yours will too.

Bunever yours,

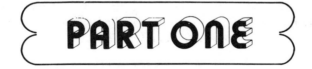

PART ONE

Bunnetics—
The Theory Behind
the Behind

While there are many good exercise books, most of them dedicate only a couple of pages to buns, which you find under the heading of buttocks—such an ugly name for something so pretty. In *Bunnetics* you will find entire series designed specifically for buns and their surrounding areas. And rather than just have you copy what I do, I have taken meticulous care to describe *what* you are doing as well as *why*. Keeping this in mind while looking at the pictures and sketches will help you to work correctly. In addition, some of the exercises will have instructions for postural alignment, the most commonly overlooked factor in exercises and the key to their effectiveness. Read the directions carefully.

If you are determined and do the exercises regularly, you will indeed see a change within a short period of time. But if you are like many people whose good intentions far exceed their determination, you may try the exercises only a couple of times and see no change. Discouraged, you may set the book on the bookcase where it will sit alone and unread until another impulsive purchase gives it a companion. I have taken this into account and have come up with two reasons why this won't happen with this book.

First—Bunnetics works on the theory that knowing and understanding one's anatomy while executing a combination of isometric, isotonic, and basic dance movements will bring about rapid muscle tone, firmness, and coordination without expending unnecessary energy. Learning one's anatomy could take forever, but the familiarization with those parts that directly relate to the buns will take just a few minutes of reading.

The second reason you won't be able to put this book on the shelf is that each exercise comes with the curse: "YOU'D BETTER FINISH ME BEFORE YOU REST, OR YOUR * * * WILL NEVER BE ITS BEST."

The use of "imagined movement" found in some of the Bunnetics exercises is often employed by me in the teaching of posture and correct alignment in the dance. This method is called Ideokinesis by Dr. Lulu E. Sweigard in her book *Human Movement Potential: Its Ideokinetic Facilitation,* which has also been a valuable reference and inspiration in the writing of *Bunnetics.* The images created by your mind (Ideo) while executing a series of movements (Kinesis) are, for the most part, the basis of the warm-up exercises.

To make any changes in your buns, you must first know and visualize which muscles, specifically in the abdomen, lower back, and thighs, will contribute to changes and ultimately a new shape. In the chapter "Buns Are Muscles," you will familiarize yourself with your set of buns through brief explanations and drawings of the muscles we will be working with to achieve our goals. Thus, before you start your program you will know the *why's* and the *what's* of each exercise.

For those readers who might be five to ten pounds overweight, the chapter "Putting Fat Behind You" is a must. For those between ten and twenty pounds over, "The Unconscious Gulping" and "The Disaster Food Diary" will be of additional help. But regardless of what weight problem you may have, keep in mind that there is no exercise plan that will allow you to lose weight at a speed that will satisfy your ardent desire to be "skinnier" without a change in your eating habits.

Adam's Seat vs. Eve's Sofa

I think what really happened between those two is that Eve was jealous of Adam's buns and also resented having to schlepp all over the jungle looking for three large leaves when he could get away with just a small one. "What's his secret?" she wondered. Then she saw him looking at an apple. In her innocence she thought this fruit was the cause for his little hips and tight buns. "What is good for the goose is good for the gander" a little snake whispered, and so she bit away! Her life changed, but her hips stayed the same.

The same jealousy has remained unchanged throughout the evolution of the sexes, but now we attribute bun shape differences to anatomy. Today we know the anatomical difference lies mainly in the pelvis, which at birth is the same in both sexes. As we grow, however, Eve's flares out, making the distance between its two edges much wider than Adam's. The development of androgen, a male sex hormone, is said to contribute to the development of his pelvis, and the addition of a thicker layer of fat forms the curves around hers. It is these curves that are harder for her to shape than for him.

Perhaps if both of them had stuck to eating just apples, today we wouldn't have such fluctuations in fat deposits. Eve has more isolated ones, but hers are of greater magnitude. She has a band of fat cells that runs from under the breasts down to the lower abdomen, or pubis, and even a larger accumulation covering the buns, hips, and halfway down the side of the leg. As if this were not enough, she has another band in front of each thigh.

Adam is a little more fortunate, for his fat deposits, although more widely distributed, are of less density than Eve's. His run from under the breasts down to the pubis, with more accumulation in the front of the stomach and the sides of the body—like an apron of fat. But his accumulation over the buns is thinner and does not cover as large a territory. It seldom gets to the sides or front of the thigh.

There are people who have more than an average number of deposits of these fat cells (or adipose tissue) covering the buns. This is called *steatophiga*, and through studies of African tribes—where it is commonly seen—it has been labeled a genetic factor. In fact, big hips and buns are generally genetically influenced, especially from mother to daughter. That is not to say that proper exercise and nutrition, especially in the teen years, cannot control this—they can.

Pregnancy is also a time when women show a greater increase of fat cells and deposits. Here again is a reason why many obstetricians recommend constant exercise up to the time of delivery, and shortly after. I have known many dancers who have practically left the ballet bar, made a grand jeté into the delivery room, and twirled right back to class.

With diet a person can reduce the size of his or her fat cells, but not the number. Only through surgery (a lipectomy) can fat cells actually be removed. There are several surgical procedures designed to remove the fat around the buns and thighs of men and women, specifically the latter when cellulite is a problem. These operations are often performed by cosmetic surgeons. Cellulite is the accumulation of stagnating water-logged tissues on the upper thighs and buns. It is formed by the debris of fat cells which deposits itself in areas where the circulation is poor. Decades ago it was practically unknown, but as women have led progressively more sedentary lives, eat more starches and sweets, and drink more alcohol, it has become a more common affliction. Off-and-on crash diets also contribute to the problem.

Most nutritionists agree that cellulite can be prevented or remedied by increased physical activity, a balanced protein diet, and the complete elimination of starches and sweets from the diet. Some advocate all the vitamins a person can afford, especially vitamin C, which prevents capillaries from enlarging and causing bad circulation. Because my Bunnetics exercises concentrate in the use of the leg and thigh muscles, they will most definitely be beneficial to women with this problem.

There has also been a recent upsurge in the amount of plastic surgeries done to both men and women who wish to have larger buns. This operation requires the use of implants and is not recommended by the best surgeons. "Riding britches" operations (also called buttocks lifts, tucks, or contouring) are widely being requested by both sexes. They are not difficult surgical procedures, but expensive ones, and in most cases could be avoided by correct exercise. All in all, Adam and Eve would not have approved of them, but then again, they had other things to think about.

Exercise—The Controversy

There are diet doctors who do not recommend exercise. They specialize in very overweight and obese people and want their patients to concentrate on the eating plan they prescribe and nothing else. Understandable, especially when I know many people say, "Doctor, I don't know why I haven't lost more weight this week, I exercised like a dog." (Well, most dogs I know only eat once a day.) The theory that exercise makes one hungry is a fallacy. It might make you thirsty due to the loss of water, but that is only if you have worked yourself into a frenzy. "But I *do* get hungry," some of you say. My answer is, "It is all in your mind, silly." We have been conditioned to believe that exercise makes us lose weight, and we don't see anything wrong with a little snack after it. But a snack can be anywhere from a carrot to a banana split.

Well, get a hold of your britches in case this shocks you. The amount of calories we lose through intermittent exercise, that is, exercise once or twice a week, does not amount to enough energy to sap a lightning bug. In a way, those non-exercising diet doctors are quite correct, but why then are they on the golf course when we need them? If starting an exercise plan is just done to get into a tighter pair of Jordache or a sexier bikini, it's a start but not the answer. Exercise has to be part of your weekly routine. Otherwise, why struggle for such a short time? Jeans come in all sizes and summer is over before you know it.

Only when it is part of your regular schedule does exercise help burn the excess fat contained by our muscles. Exercise raises your body heat, allowing your metabolism to burn more calories throughout the day. Exercising and improper eating can easily make you even heavier, for as the muscles are worked they will turn muscle fat into hard muscle fiber, which weighs more than fat. It is even possible to increase your body size when the exercised muscles get larger and push the subcutaneous fat you haven't lost farther out. I hope this convinces you that the only way to get good buns is through proper eating *and* a well-balanced exercise program. Bunnetics is an exercise program that uses the buns as the primary beneficiary. It is not a spot-reducing program. I don't believe such a program can work. It is impossible to just isolate one area of the body without assistance from adjoining parts. In dance we have known this for centuries. We are bound together by lots of muscles, and fat belongs to the entire body, not to just one single muscle. It is not impossible, however, to work an area containing large sets of muscles, like buns and legs, whose action benefits surrounding spots such as the stomach, thighs, and hips. All Bunnetic movements are designed to work problem areas by slowly conditioning the muscles by increasing their workload through a five-week period and, when needed, decreasing the food intake.

In short this is what Bunnetics will do for you:

• Will help you turn fat-filled muscles into lean muscles.
• Will help to change your body's shape.
• Will help to develop better muscle tone, coordination, and posture.
• Will contribute to developing a higher fat-burning metabolism.

With the added help of "The Disaster Food Diary" you will also:

• Become aware of your unconscious gulping and pay attention to values of the food you eat.
• Make your own balanced eating plan.
• Reduce body size.

The two combined will:

• Help you change body size and shape.
• Give your buns a better casing.
• Make you smile a few times.

Here's another Pre-Bun exercise. Let's rehearse it now.

"The Ripple"

POSTURAL ALIGNMENT

If you are sitting on a straight-back chair (the only type you should have if you sit a lot), lean your torso forward so as to form a 45° angle with your thighs, which should be parallel but not together. Both knees should be in a direct line away from the hip bones. Put the book down for a second and place hands on both thighs. Round your back a little and bring your chin down to touch the chest. Please read again before doing. Now.

Through 10 slow counts you are going to start by squeezing your buns together then continuing the contraction to the lower stomach, diaphragm, rib cage, torso, chest, and, finally, as your back and neck straighten (and you sit up erect), pushing the shoulders down while pressing your hands on your thighs.

COUNTS

1	Tighten your buns
2	Continue the contraction to the lower stomach
3	The diaphragm (start straightening the spine)
4	Rib cage (continue to straighten slowly)
5	Torso and chest (finally straightening completely)
6	Neck and shoulders (keeping back straight)
7, 8, 9, 10	Hold position for 4 counts.
	Relax and do one more time, then continue to read.

Sedentary = Bunnentary

Webster's dictionary defines the word sedentary as "stationary, requiring much sitting." I define it as "bunnentary, requiring much resting on your buns." Oh, I know there are a lot of terrific looking people with office jobs who manage to keep their buns in shape in spite of sitting all day. But those buns don't get that way by themselves.

Exercising your muscles above their normal capacity is the only way to keep them fat free and firm enough to maintain a good figure. On the other hand, you can also find people whose work requires a lot of physical activity, and they still manage to get fat. The reason is that their work does not use the full capacity of their muscle power. It is "busy work" and not to be confused with exercise. Their muscles get accustomed to the required activity and are able to perform their functions with a gradual decrease of energy expenditure. This is clearly seen with dancers during the first weeks of a show. Everyone loses weight while their muscles learn and perfect the routine, and after the show opens they tend to regain the lost pounds and even add a few extra. The hardships of learning and rehearsal become routine through the repetition of performance. Constantly busy housewives with large families are another example. They might be dead at the end of the day, but their muscles have been used only to a small percentage of their work-load capacity. Due to the larger unused percentage, fat accumulates, and after reaching a saturation point (which depends on the individual's body frame) the excess is stored outside the muscle. This new deposit takes the form of adipose tissue or subcutaneous fat, which is what you see and feel. Getting too large is not an overnight occurrence. Long before it shows on the outside a lot has been happening in the inside.

Stop. Do one *Ripple*

As we get older and strive for personal and financial growth, it's easy to become bunnentary. It is a direct result of comfort. Besides, our society is continuously flooded with inventions designed to make us burn less energy. Bunnentary temptations are all over. The location where you live or work has tremendous impact on your fat-burning process. In large cities like New York and Chicago people do a great deal for walking. In New York there are times of the day when you move faster than the cars, and that burns energy, and energy burns fat. In smaller cities or suburban neighborhoods, cars are your buns' (big ones) best friend.

For instance, when I visit my parents in Florida and go to the market, which is just five blocks away, I get in the car. After thirty leisurely minutes of pushing a cart through aisles of overweight Bermuda shorts I drive back, stop at the Dairy Queen, and without getting out of the car I can enjoy my Jumbo Rocky Road shake. No wonder when I get home it becomes much harder to get out of the car than it was to get in. All that sugar and air goes straight to my butt. In New York, I run to the market, speed through the aisles, and then run home praying that when I turn the corner no one will steal the groceries right out of my hands. The running and the fear burn even more energy.

Speaking of burning energy, it is time for:

The Tenderizer

Rock back and forth on the seat of your chair twenty times, tightening your buns every time you go back and releasing every time you go forward. Then reverse, tightening when you go forward and releasing when you go back. If anyone is watching don't stop, but don't smile either. Try it a couple of times.

But back to where I started. As we get older and more settled, good living is expressed with values different from the ones we had in our book-carrying years. Back then we weren't allowed to stay up late, smoke, or drink martinis, and sports activities were something we did while our parents watched. Fortunately, times are changing. We might still be a youth-oriented society, but more people are now recognizing that children are not the only ones who need exercise and healthy habits. If you are part of those who think that exercise is a *luxury* for the "old," it's time to change. Being young is thinking young, and staying young is keeping fit, and the tighter your buns are the younger you will feel. Proper eating and correct exercise will firm up buns and erase wrinkles. You can bet on it!

Putting Fat Behind You

Are you overweight? Probably. Reports indicate that the majority of Americans are, and if reports do not impress you, then go out the door and take a good look. We are surrounded by fat!

Overweight is a national problem and has become big business. How many times have you said you're going on a diet and carted your fat to the bookstore in search of the miracle "pounds-off" book? You probably lost more weight looking for such a book than you would have after the first week of following its instructions. A diet book is not the answer. YOU HAVE TO CHANGE YOUR EATING HABITS IF YOU WANT TO LOSE WEIGHT. I know it and you do too, but somehow we must read it to believe it.

How do you know if you are overweight? Well there are several ways. One is the "pinch" method, which you can do by grasping a fold of skin at the back of the upper arm between thumb and forefinger. If your grab gives you between one-half to one-inch thickness, you are fine. More than an inch, you are fat. Less than one-half inch, you are a rail. Then there is the method where you place a ruler on your stomach along the midline. It should touch both the ribs and the pelvic area. (If you can't find either area, don't even bother with the ruler—you are definitely fat.) My favorite method is standing naked in front of the mirror. The mirror does not lie.

There are, of course, more scientific methods of determining excess weight, but for our purposes a look in the mirror or the pinch test is enough. Nevertheless, if you find you are 25 pounds or more over your "desirable weight," a visit to your physician is a must, especially if you haven't had a complete medical examination in the last two years. ("The Disaster Food Diary," page 122, includes a discussion of "desirable weight.")

Overweight is without question a very controversial subject and one of constant study and research. Various tables of recommended weights are under constant criticism for their shortcomings. What is body frame? Isn't a person of large frame but average height bound to weigh more than a person of small frame and the same height? Doesn't a person's profession have anything to do with their ideal weight?

Dr. Jean Mayers, well-known nutritionist and author, states in a recent article for the New York *Daily News* that once a person is fully grown (mid-twenties) any weight gained is bound to be added fat. He continues on to say that if you were slim and in good health at that age, your weight at that time is a good target to shoot for now. If you can't remember that far back, then sticking to the tables might be your choice. Dr. Mayers says, "Extreme obesity is, of course, easy to identify—all you have to do is look." You see, the mirror wins again!

The mirror, the dancer's curse, has an unbelievable memory bank. It immediately reflects a bad performance and rewards its correction with a reminder of the former "flop." The same is true for weight. When you are fat, the mirror insults you; and when you get skinnier, it still makes you think you are fat.

The present diet rush clearly shows a growing concern about too much weight. Unfortunately, it is impossible to go to sleep fat and wake up skinny. At the same time, if all the people who vouch that they are on a diet really were, carrot stick stands would have replaced pizza shops a long time ago. Most folks go on diets to lose weight quickly, regardless of consequences and medical warnings. The smart way to lose weight (as we all know) is to lose it gradually while permanently changing eating habits. If you need to lose weight, watching what you eat while learning about food is not being on a diet. It is, however, being smart. I not only watch *what* I eat, but *when* I eat, and *how much* I eat. The phrase "You can never be too rich or too thin" hangs over my bathroom scale. I confess that there are times when I must pig-out. Why not? It feels good when I do. But I make sure these binges don't happen too frequently (primarily reserved for holidays) and ensure they are followed by short, suffering periods of food celibacy. From my own studies and from hundreds of questionnaires given to dancers and dance enthusiasts, I have compiled "The Dancer's Skinny Eating" tips, which appears at the end of this book.

Feeling unhappy or depressed is your stomach's best friend. Once, in one of my depressed periods when I could not dance due to an injury I sustained lifting a fat ballerina (we do have them), I climbed up to 175 pounds in less than two months. For someone 5′ 8″ who always hovers around the 145 pound mark, that was *heavy*. You talk about buns and gut! Mine sort of fused together to form a very impressive Flipper look-alike. For me, depression and ice cream go hand-in-hand. During this period the trading stock in Häagen Daaz, Manhattan's favorite ice cream, must have risen 6 points.

When my doctor gave the go-ahead to start dancing, I was too embarrassed to go into a dance class. You see, dancers must go to class every day to keep the body in shape. Class is our daily Waterloo. I went—but not before stopping at a Capezio's dance-wear shop and buying every dance outfit in black I could get my hands on. It did not help. When you wear all black, people know you are hiding something. They avoid looking you straight in the eye, but never hesitate to look at your bulges. So what did I do?

Sorry, not before you do 2 **Shifters,** 1 **Clincher,** and 1 **Dimpler.** Now you can read on.

Well, I changed my strategy and wore light-colored clothes that would show my newly acquired rolls. Whenever I looked at myself in the mirror I knew I had to do something about them. It was sickening! I had to lose weight fast. I knew I could not stop eating, especially when after resting for so long, dance classes tired me out. Just like many of you, I went searching for a diet book and accidentally ended up browsing through a book on nutrition, C. Robinson's *Normal and Therapeutic Nutrition*. It changed my life!

I decided that if I knew more about the foods that would allow me to lose weight and still maintain my energy, I could make my own diet. I set out to do some studying, and after years of absence rediscovered the Public Library. I wasn't totally ignorant about the subject of nutrition. Next to dance, weight and food are a dancer's favorite subjects. I must say, however, that the more conflicting theories and statistics I read, the more confused I got. I realized it was going to take more than just a couple of hours of reading but, if necessary, I was willing to bring my ballet bar and bed to the Library.

As my research progressed, my understanding of the nutritional process improved and things started to fall into place. It was simple. I had been swimming in a pool of sugar and starches that was rapidly overflowing the amount of calories I was burning every day. It did not take me long to realize what my next move had to be. I went home and threw away my sweet tooth by burying my sugar bowl in the back yard, feeding all my cookies and candies to my love birds, dumping the ice cream on my plants, and yes, taking up smoking! In less than two months I was back to my normal weight. My plants were greener and fatter than ever, my love birds wouldn't look at each other and ended up in separate cages, and I am still smoking and have been trying to quit for three years. If you are overweight, you can do it too. Eighty-six that sweet tooth! Only *you* can decide when and if you really wish to change your eating habits. And while you think about it:

The Lazy Sit-Up (Part One)

POSTURAL ALIGNMENT

Sit up straight with feet flat on the floor and about 6 inches apart. Let your arms hang free along the sides of the body.

Without tightening your buns muscles at all, lift your right thigh from the seat of the chair then extend the leg as you incline your torso forward and over the thigh.

Make sure that your back stays straight and your arms relaxed alongside. Return to starting position.

Do the same with the left thigh.

Alternate with right and left to a total of 10 repetitions, 5 with the right, and 5 with the left.

Relax and do not repeat.

(Part Two)

POSTURAL ALIGNMENT

Place both hands alongside the chair with fingers pointing toward the floor but thumbs resting on seat of chair. In that position squeeze your buns real tight and lift both thighs up from the seat of the chair while pressing down on your arms—keep your shoulders down. You may want to lean back as your thighs go up. Fight this by pushing your straight back forward with the use of your arms against the chair.

Hold for 10 counts. Relax and do not repeat.

Fats Are More Fun Behind
Other People's Behinds . . .

Gaining weight is easy. Getting rid of it can be a pain. There are many different reasons why people gain weight. In the chapter "The Unconscious Gulping" I will try to elaborate on a few of them. But since I want to get you through this whole section and ready for Buns One, I will just take the two main reasons for gaining weight. They are ignorance and too much of the wrong food. Food in our country is so much more plentiful and varied than in other countries that we take its nutritional value for granted. Much research has been done during the last few years by government agencies, nutritionists, and physicians to help us know and evaluate what we eat. I have the feeling most of it ends up unread at the Public Library. Their books on the subject still have that fresh-off-the-press look.

America is a youth- and sex-oriented society, and the word "nutrition" has little sex appeal. Although most popular magazines have great articles written by distinguished people, we often pass them by in search of the pictures of the beautiful men and women whose clothes, hair, looks, and life styles we want to emulate with our fat bodies. I think that if the Food and Nutrition Board would make a list entitled "Recommended Daily Sexual Food Allowance" it would become the nation's best seller. Fat chance, but more people would eat better.

"You are what you eat" is a statement that I frequently read. Food gives us the nutrients we convert to energy in order to love, grow, and get fat. Nutrients are materials that nourish the body. They have three primary functions: fuel for energy, the building and upkeep of body tissues, and providing the materials to regulate the body processes. They are divided into five major groups: carbohydrates, proteins, fats, vitamins, and minerals.

If you are overweight, learning about these nutrients is your first task toward accomplishing the desired results from Bunnetics.

CARBOHYDRATES

Research has proven that no food substance is composed of just one nutrient. When we speak of a carbohydrate food, we mean one containing more carbohydrate than any other nutrient. Carbohydrates are the easiest on our pocketbook and are our major source of energy for brain function and muscular exertion. They are essential to the digestive process since they assist in the assimilation of other foods, and are the body's major source of glucose, our life-sustaining fuel. Nutritionists suggest that 1 gram of carbohydrate for every 3 pounds of "ideal weight" be eaten daily in order to maintain proper body function.

Unfortunately, many people associate carbohydrate foods exclusively with sweets, pastries, and starchy foods. These carbohydrates are "empty ones," lacking in the nutrients we need. When taken in excess they can't be used by the body and are thus stored as fat. After ingestion they are immediately converted into glucose, and this rapid delivery to the bloodstream activates the release of insulin in large amounts. Thus, the suggestion "Eat sugar for quick energy." Remember that what goes up comes down. In this case with a crash!

"Complete" carbohydrates—such as those found in cereals, and fresh fruits and vegetables and their juices—provide the nutrients we need and are less burdensome to the body's digestive process. They are broken down into glucose at a slower rate, resulting in a weaker, but continuous flow of insulin. This allows the digestive process to properly distribute glucose to the building tissues of the body.

White processed sugar, the Wicked Witch of the Fatsos, is the worst of the empty carbohydrates. It has no vitamins, no minerals, no proteins, and no fat. As stated before, it is solely a provider of quick energy. But you should know that the same, and more prolonged, energy can be obtained from better and more nutritious food sources. The average consumption of sugar is about 102 pounds per person per year. That is like carrying around your own Space Shuttle all day. Even more important, you should know that sugar is the number one B-vitamin-depleting factor because the body, in its effort to convert sugar (sucrose) into glucose, uses up a great amount of the body's supply of this vitamin. You never need to think about not getting enough sugar. Even meat and liver contain starch, which is digested into glucose. In fact, about 65 percent of the food you eat is turned to sugar. Like me, you can bury the sugar bowl and still obtain a plentiful share of it.

All in all, good carbohydrates have a very important function in our daily diet. They are our main source of energy and are relatively rich in other nutrients.

PROTEINS

Proteins are required by people of all ages. About 20 percent of our body is protein, with most of it concentrated in the form of muscle. It is also found in bone cartilage, organs, and endocrine glands. Eggs, milk, yogurt, meat, and fish are the best animal sources of protein, and beans, peas, cereals, and nuts the best plant sources.

Proteins are made up of building units called amino acids. There are 22 amino acids, and these synthesize the hundreds of proteins used for countless body functions, chiefly the building of body tissues like muscle, heart, skin, and hair. Of all the amino acids, eight are considered "essential" because they can't be manufactured by the body and must be acquired from first-class protein foods.

Nutritionists agree that most people do not get enough protein, either through ignorance in selecting a good diet or because of financial reasons. (Protein foods are generally the most expensive.) It is said that to maintain a balanced diet we need about 0.8 gram of protein per kilogram of body weight (1 kg. = 2.2 lbs.). In simpler terms, a man of 154 pounds would need about 56 grams daily, and 44 grams would be necessary for a woman weighing about 120 pounds. A general misconception is that muscular work increases the requirement for protein intake. Actually, body size determines that. In even simpler terms, if you are built like a house, you need more to move your foundation around. But protein should not be your primary source of energy. It should be eaten along with, and not to the exclusion of, carbohydrates, so that your body can use it for the building of body tissues, leaving carbohydrates for energy. Otherwise, the body must use protein for both functions, which is neither efficient nor inexpensive.

Now we come to fat, but not before we give the technical part of our brain a rest and activate all those fat cells in our buns.

Do Two *Lazy Sit-Ups* (**Part One and Part Two**)

FAT

If the name of this very important nutrient doesn't tell you anything, then perhaps knowing that fat is the major source of energy stored by your body as "adipose tissue" will. Adipose cells are found all over your body, either singly or in small groups and especially in loose connective tissue. Needless to say, we require a certain amount of fat in our body. As a matter of fact, half of the body's deposit of fat is found right under the skin, serving as a protective shield from the environment. Skinny people will feel cold weather much more than really fat ones, but skinnies have the consolation of knowing that a fur coat for an overweight person will have to have more skins to get around all that bulk, and thus cost more.

Most foods contain fat, but few are made exclusively of it. Fat is divided into animal and vegetable fat. The animal groups are meat; fish, poultry, milk and its products, and egg yolks. The vegetable groups are margarine, seeds, vegetable oils, and some vegetables and fruits. Fats do have some very important roles. They carry the vitamins A, D, E, and K throughout the body, and allow proteins to be used for their more important function—the building of body tissues—instead of being consumed strictly for energy. Nutritional research experts, in their constant experimentation to provide us with solutions to the problems of the worldwide feeding and overpopulation, have tried feeding rats with a fat-free diet. Ever see a skinny rat? Because of the diet these creatures did not grow properly, and developed kidney and skin disorders. What a shame!

Those of you wanting to shed a few pounds should realize that meals containing some fat will stay with you longer because they are digested and absorbed at a slower pace. Gayelord Hauser, who has spent most of his life instructing people in the benefits of nutrition, and whose books I found to be among the best on the subject, states that Americans consume 40 to 50 percent of their calories in hard fats. No wonder high cholesterol is found among so many of our senior citizens. Mr. Hauser recommends the use of certain vegetable oils, as opposed to the more common hydrogenated oils, as the best to stimulate the burning of stored fat. Safflower, sunflower, and poppyseed oil rate among the most frequently recommended. I, for one, try to have a daily spoonful of safflower oil (in salad dressing, for instance) and believe it does wonders for my hair and skin.

Unfortunately, fatty food is good-tasting food. Mothers, our stomachs' very own Florence Nightingales, are always telling us, "You need to put more meat on those bones." They use this as an excuse to demonstrate their cooking expertise. My mother shops every day for three months before I visit so that when I arrive for a stay, four times a year, she can dump the whole thing in my stomach in a week's time—though as a nurse, she knows better. But what can I do? My bones and my buns just love her, and I do too!

VITAMINS AND MINERALS

Today, not even Carter has as many pills as there are stores dedicated exclusively to selling vitamins. My advice is that you spend a little time doing some research before you take all kinds of pills that might do you more harm than good. I have a bunch of pill-o-maniac friends who must spend a substantial part of the day counting and taking vitamins. I stick to the same multivitamin that I have used for years.

I think it is safe to say that if you follow a well-balanced diet, you will get all the nutrients necessary, including vitamins and minerals, and still be able to lose your excess weight and keep it off. Having a balanced diet is easily accomplished by following the food guide, *Food for Fitness, a Daily Food Guide,* developed by the Institute of Home Economics of the Agricultural Research Service. This simple guide divides all food into four major groups: milk group, vegetable group, meat group, and bread-cereal group. It recommends the proper serving amounts for each group that a person should include in his daily diet for well-balanced meals. These amounts are:

Milk Group	— 2 cups
Vegetable Group	— 2 cups (4 servings)
Meat Group	— 2 servings (8 oz.)
Bread-Cereal	— 4 servings

Although this is a good, general guideline, it is essential to know the nutritional value of the foods in each group so that well-balanced selections and substitutions can be made. Where there is a will there is a way, and if you are determined to lose that extra weight without having to go on starvation diets, or the ones where your stomach must endure being a water-filled bubble, you will find the way.

The word "servings" has its shortcomings, one being that it does not have the same meaning for everyone. For instance, the average serving of meat or fish is considered to be about a quarter of a pound. A serving of fruit or vegetable should be in the neighborhood of half a cup. For most of us who do not eat at home the majority of the time and who are not about to carry a cup with us all day, the concept of "serving" does present a problem. In that case, this is what you should do. When you are home, pay attention to the suggested measurements and keep a visual impression of the sizes of the portions. Then try to stick to them when eating out. It only takes a little discipline, which I know is easier said than done.

Whatever happened to *calories?* Don't worry, they are not dead. They are indestructible. Actually, it is your body that can easily be destroyed by an excess of them, and because of their importance I felt I would leave them for the end to create a lasting impression. But first, you have been reading for quite a while, and it is time to give those buns a rest, a stretch, and a hug. Time to stand up! Here comes

The Sexy Runner

(NOTE: If you are not at home or by yourself, I would suggest you try *The Ripple* instead.) This is one of the best exercises for the buns and the entire thigh, and it helps to tighten up the lower abdomen, too (but it has also been known to arouse pets).

POSTURAL ALIGNMENT

Stand up with both feet parallel and about 6 inches apart. While still maintaining a parallel position move your left foot forward so that its heel is slightly in front of the right foot, and your body's weight is between both feet. Now, flex both knees, and then raise the heel of the left foot from the floor as high as it will go. The weight on your left foot is now supported by the ball of the foot and toes. Let your arms rest alongside the body.

Now: Bring your pelvis forward and upward toward the stomach while tightening your buns and thighs. Relax and release. Repeat again for a total of 5 times, then change positions by placing the right foot forward and doing the same.

CALORIES

A lot of people speak of calories without actually knowing what they really are. I get a kick when I see people talking about skipping a meal because they are watching their calories. In the meantime they are gorging on a slice of pizza with half the Italian meat market spread all over it. Calories are a unit of heat. They measure the amount of energy produced by different foods when processed by the body. Some foods are richer than others in the amount of calories their processing gives, but calories are the same whether they come from proteins, carbohydrates, or fats. This is how it works:

$$1 \text{ gm. of Carbohydrate} \quad - \quad 4 \text{ calories}$$
$$1 \text{ gm. of Protein} \quad = \quad 4 \text{ calories}$$
$$1 \text{ gm. of Fat} \quad = \quad 9 \text{ calories}$$

Our body is a constantly burning furnace. Even when it is in a state of rest (called Basal Metabolism) it is burning off heat, a form of energy. And this heat is measured in calories. A calorie is the amount of heat it takes to raise the temperature of one pint of water 8° F, or 1 kg. of water 1° C. (The calorie used in metabolic figures is the "large calorie," which is 1,000 times larger than the "small calorie" used in physics.) The amount of activity a person engages in determines the number of calories burned above the Basal Metabolism. (Basal Metabolism is covered further in "The Disaster Food Diary.") The "average" woman needs about 2,000 calories and the "average" man needs 2,700.

Though excess weight increases as we get older, the amount of calories required decreases. That is why we must regulate our intake of them as we get closer to that Social Security check. A younger person following the recommendations of the four-food-group guide will be getting about 1,200 calories, thus having some space for a certain amount of desserts. An older person has to be much more careful.

When you intake more calories than your body needs, you gain weight; less calories than you need, you lose. Since the body also requires specific amounts of all three basic nutrients, weight loss through a reduction in calories must be accompanied by a method for properly balancing the nutrients. This takes a little bit of simple mathematics and is also covered in "The Disaster Food Diary" and the "Dance Bag Diet."

A person who is physically active will burn more calories than the average bunnentary person but still gain weight if he overdoes his or her caloric intake. At the same time, an athlete could very well be overweight, according to the weight tables, but not fat. An athlete's body gets used to the amount of pounding it receives and after a while it seems to require it. And because of the reversibility factor of overworked muscles, when it does not get a daily workout —due to injury or even a short vacation—it revolts in the form of added fat.

Learn to select and combine from the four-food-group those things you enjoy the most. The choice is endless. That's all you need to change your eating habits and allow those presently cloud-covered buns to come out through the clear blue yonder. Well, maybe that's not all. In one of her television specials actress Shirley MacLaine talked of the dancer's Four D's. They are Desire, Determination, Drive, and Discipline. Although I am biased, I think those Four D's say a lot. If you need to lose weight, use their message and your own common sense.

Buns Are Muscles

Buns, with the help from other muscles, form the supportive frame that controls posture, movement, coordination, and balance. These muscles lie at the back of the pelvis, which is at the base of the trunk. Not only is this the area where the center of gravity lies, but it is probably the most important area of the body for movement and balance. Thus, the phrase, "Move your ass." Muscles are made up of a rich supply of blood and nerves, and a functional unit called the muscle fibers, which are wrapped in thin sheets of tissue bound together by more tissues that vary in thickness, density, and fat according to their requirements and location in the body. Muscles constitute 40 to 50 percent of the body's weight, and come in three types: cardiac, as in the heart; smooth, as in the stomach; and skeletal, which allow for the movement of the entire body or parts of the body. There are approximately 600 skeletal muscles. Some are external, and—depending on the individual's physical development—can be visibly distinguished. These would include: the Rectus Abdominis, the Gluteus Maximus, and the Latissimus Dorsi, for instance. Others are internal and intermediary, like the Psoas Major or the Gluteus Minimus, and as such are hard or impossible to find regardless of physique. The Bunnetics exercises will focus on nineteen of these muscles, whether singularly or in functional groups. The majority of them will be external muscles.

Bun size depends not only on the size of the muscle fibers and the amount of connective tissue that binds these fibers, but on genetic factors, the size of the pelvis (broader for women than for men), and on the amount of subcutaneous fat that surrounds the buns. In some cases there can be almost twice as much fat as there is muscle. The strength of your bun muscles is judged by their degree of contracting force. Thus, big buns are not necessarily strong buns. The only way to strengthen them, as it is with all muscles, is by continuous and increasing amounts of work (the Overload Principle).

For the average person, a regular schedule of light and continuous exercise, such as the Bunnetics program, promotes better
circulation of blood to the muscles, as well as firmness, tone, and
coordination. Weight lifting, long a favorite way for men, and more
recently for women, to change their body shape without having to
be active sports people, is another form of exercise. It does have
some drawbacks, however. The most obvious is overdevelopment
of the muscles, which produces bulky contractile fibers. This does
give a strong and well-defined muscled look (boundness) but at
the sacrifice of elasticity, suppleness, and range of movement. Regardless of what form of exercise we give our muscles, it must be
realized that their activity depends solely on our nervous system.
Stated another way, the contractions of the muscles, be they isometric (contraction of muscles without movement), isotonic (contraction with movement), or isokinetic (movement with a controlled
resistance, as in the use of exercise machines), cannot take place
without the impulse or command from the brain.

Skeletal muscles have odd characteristics, various functions, and
mixed personalities. They are irritable, responding to command;
contractile, changing shape by becoming shorter or thicker; stretch-
able, being able to extend; and elastic, returning to their original
form after stretching. Functionally, they work like members of
Congress as agonists, or prime movers; antagonists, movers in the
opposite direction; synergists, preventing undesired movements;
and stabilizers, trying to maintain order despite strong opposition.
Their personalities vary tremendously. Some are bitchy, like the
ones in the face when you get angry; some are sort of floppy, like
those in the back of the upper arm found in many women and in
most mother-in-laws; some are sexy, like those . . . well, they vary
according to what makes you tick. But regardless of their various
qualities, they are all very gregarious and group themselves into either voluntary muscles, which do what you tell them to do, or in-
voluntary muscles, to which your commands go totally unheard unless you are a Yogi.

Officially, they have odd tongue-twisting names given by the
Greeks. Wouldn't you know it! For ease of memorization I have
taken the liberty of renaming some of the muscles that will take
part in our daily Bunnetic exercises. These muscles are the ones
that will help you attain the muscle tone needed to develop firmer
buns, a tighter stomach, shaplier thighs, and a better posture.

The Bunnetic exercises are executed in two stages, the warm-ups and the exercises. The warm-ups, which remain the same throughout the program, depend in part on your mind's ability to create moving pictures. Be it through visualization, fantasy, association, or comparison, with the added assistance of *imagined movement,* you will perform them with a minimum amount of energy and maximum degree of efficiency. *Imagined movement* means forming a picture in your mind of the mechanics of the movement before you do it; visualizing what is happening while you do it, often with the help of another image or comparison; and clearing your mind in preparation for the next movement. Each Bunnetic warm-up is formed by imagery, action, contraction, and rest. The second stage, the exercises, are a series of simple movements with increased workloads over a five-week period.

To perform all stages effectively, a basic knowledge of the primary functions and location of the muscles at work is essential. Thus, the following sketches and the descriptions of muscle groups will need more than one reading, although as Bunnetics progresses into a daily routine the given names of the muscles and specific movements will become second nature. It is important to note that these descriptions are just a means to facilitate your visualization or imagery before their execution so that *you feel the action from the inside out* rather than as a reflex action to a picture or written instruction. As Agatha Christie's famous detective Hercule Poirot would say, "You let the mind's little gray cells help you solve the mystery." It is the brain's command through your nervous system that moves those muscles.

Meet the Bunnetic Stars

Such important personalities cannot be introduced without a little bit of theatricality. So curtain up! Holding center stage under the main spotlight, "The Tuschy Trio," your buns!

Your buns and hips are formed by the Gluteus Maximus, or "Biggie" (its union card stage name). The Maximus muscles (one on each side) are the ones you admire the most, and are the most powerful extensors of the thigh. The Gluteus Medius, or "Tiny Buns," help to give shape to your hips by partly surrounding the hip bones as well as rotating the thigh outward and inward. He is

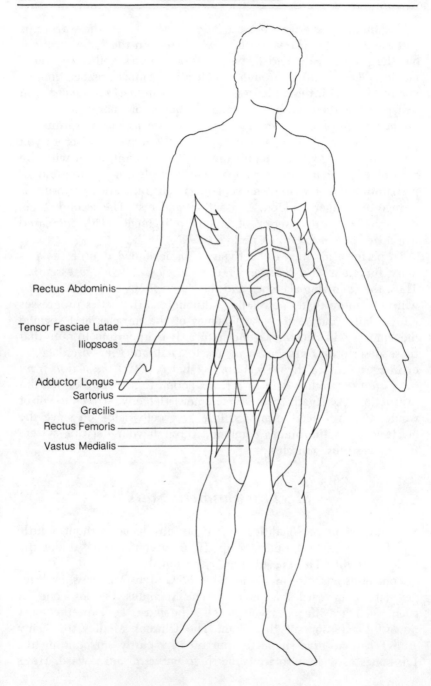

Rectus Abdominis

Tensor Fasciae Latae

Iliopsoas

Adductor Longus

Sartorius

Gracilis

Rectus Femoris

Vastus Medialis

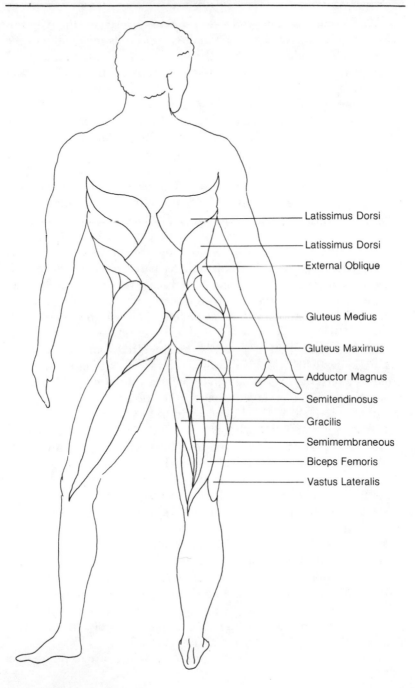

Latissimus Dorsi

Latissimus Dorsi

External Oblique

Gluteus Medius

Gluteus Maximus

Adductor Magnus

Semitendinosus

Gracilis

Semimembraneous

Biceps Femoris

Vastus Lateralis

the dancy one of the group and always upstages the Gluteus Minimus, which lies deep inside and, therefore, is impossible to see or feel. Together they sing their theme song "Love Me or Lift Me," which was a sensation among plastic surgeons before Bunnetics was developed.

And now our talented supporting cast.

Looking upward, or upstage, and to either side from center stage we have the Latissimus Dorsi, or "Lats." This widely acclaimed ensemble help to give that envious V shape we see on swimmers. The Lats connect the upper arm to the spinal column and to the back of the pelvis right above the buns. They are used any time the arms exert a downward push or the body is lifted by the arms.

No show can take place without a producer, a director, and a stage manager. We'll find them by moving around to the front of the body (the trunk). In that order they are the Psoas Major, the Rectus Abdominis, and the Iliopsoas. As part of management their work is to be felt and not seen. The Psoas Major, where filet mignon comes from (so typical of producers) is a major flexor of the trunk and most important for the development of good posture. It is one of the internal muscles that cannot be seen or felt. The Rectus Abdominis ("Mini") moves the spine front and back. It also lets us know who is a beer drinker, and its size and degree of firmness guard the abdominal cavity where your stomach is hidden. When it comes to our stage manager, the Iliopsoas, it can be safely said that practically nothing moves without its assistance.

And who is running the lights? The External Obliques, which I named "Ester" after my widowed love bird. They run from the side of the body around to the front and help to form the so-called "Love Handles," though most people who have them hate them because they are hard to tone and even harder to get rid of as we get older. While Mini flexes the spine forward and back, Ester rotates it from side to side.

And a 5-6-7. Give me music! To the orchestra pit!

The muscles of the thigh are definitely most important to the Bunnetic movements. They are going to be used as the rhythmic lever for the majority of our body movements, and just as an orchestra has four main sections—the woodwind, the brass, the string, and the percussion—the thigh is also divided in an equal number—the front, back, inside, and outside.

In the front we have the Quadriceps, which are composed of

four large separate muscles, three of which are partially united to each other. They are the Rectus Femoris, the Vastus Lateralis, the Vastus Medialis, and the Vastus Intermedius. You can lose weight by just pronouncing them. Like woodwind instruments, together they perform the same function of blowing into life the flexing[1] of the thigh and extension[2] of the knee. We'll just call them "Quads." Also in the front and running over the Quads to the inside of the knee we find the Sartorius. This muscle, who gets his name from a long line of tailors, is the longest muscle we have and is our musical director. It rotates the thigh outward when the knee is flexed.

On the side of the thigh we have "Tessie," our main percussionist, whose real-life name is Tensor Fasciae Latae. This one is a frustrated dancer and loves to do the cancan. Its main function is to rotate and abduct[3] the thigh, a movement typical of that French dance.

The inside of the thigh, our brass section, gives us our main adductor[4] muscle group: the Gracilis which adducts and flexes the thigh and the leg; the Adductor Longus, which crosses one thigh over the other; and the Adductor Magnus, the strongest of this group, which holds the trunk erect and also helps to incline it forward.

Last in our muscular overture is the string section, which is properly called the Hamstring group. They are the Semitendinosus, the Semimembranosus, and the Biceps Femoris. The Ham's primary function is to bend the knee, but it also rotates the leg and with the help of the adductors extends the leg at the hip joint (the femoral joint).

Counting them individually they come to nineteen, a good-size musical play even by Broadway standards. Some of their names will appear throughout the descriptions of many of the exercises to help you know which muscles you are working. You must remember that the actions of muscles are not individual, since skeletal muscles often share their areas of attachment (be it bone, liga-

---

[1] *flexion:* decreasing the angle between a joint and the center line of the body (the midline)

[2] *extension:* the reverse action of flexion

[3] *abduct:* draws away from the body's midline

[4] *adduct:* draws toward body's midline

ments, or skin) with other muscles.[5] So even though these nineteen individual muscles, or muscle groups (as in the case of the Quads, the Hams, or the Adductors) are selected as the main tools to our movements, any muscle action that focuses on them will put into play many other muscles. Which ones and how many depend on the action and the body's position during the action. Thus, the Bunnetic exercises follow a set pattern. They start with you lying on your back; then, on both sides, followed by resting face down; and finally in various standing positions. Different starting positions activate different muscles even in similar types of movements.

By the same token, a movement's reverse action will produce a reverse function on the muscle or group of muscles being worked. For instance, in the flexing of the thigh when lying on your back, the Iliopsoas is the principal producer of that action. It is acting as an agonist, while the Gluteus Maximus is the muscle fighting the action, or antagonist. If after flexing we immediately extend, then the Gluteus becomes the agonist and the Iliopsoas the antagonist. The same movement in a standing position activates more muscles, such as the Psoas Major, the Rectus Abdominis, and most of the groups found on the standing leg.

Toning the buns, thighs, and leg muscles is not an easy achievement; it requires daily thinking and practice. For those of you who lead a rather bunnentary life and whose legs are more flabby than muscular, or who happen to be gifted with a pair of Thunder Thighs, your determination has to be very strong. Do not despair, it can be done. Of course, if your knees are bigger than your thighs and sexier than your buns, you might be in trouble. A couple of prayers might help. Perseverance and a positive mental attitude are the key to an exquisite derriere. There is no way to get around it. To make your buns rounded, firm, and sexy, the area surrounding them must be worked on. There is no point in having the buns of life hidden by Diesel-size tires on top of two oak trees and covered by a Moby Dick paunch.

---

[5] Skeletal muscles always originate in areas closer to the center of the body (the midline) and are attached (the insertion) to areas with more mobility located farther away from the center. Quite often origin and insertion are interchangeable according to the movement being executed.

The day when you look behind you and find everyone turning their heads to stare at your behind is closer than you think. Follow The Plan, and when you get those buns in shape—show them! You owe it to your buns! In other words, when you've got it . . . flaunt it!

Mirror Mirror on the Wall, Are My Buns the Worst of All?

Of course not! They might not be Snow White's, but the fact that your mirror hasn't cracked is in itself reassuring. Remember that Snow White, the world's first jogger, spent most of her time skipping through the woods, and that is good bun-building exercise.

Although all buns are unique, there are a few types that predominate. Now that we're about ready to start The Plan, figure out which category describes you.

BUMPER BUNS

(Medium to large, rather rubbery on the outside, but with strong steel muscles inside.) These are the most common type on both men and women. Those who have them don't mind hard seats. They have been known to cause severe whiplash in Latin men who just idolize them. They are the "cloud-covered" buns I spoke of earlier, and losing fat from the outside while tenderizing the inside through firming movements is the goal.

PEAR BUNS

(Medium large to immense.) They are easy to identify, and the hardest to change because they did not get like a pear overnight. They are impossible to hide even in the strongest jeans. When their owners sit down they expand so much to either side that you could rest an ashtray on one and a drink on the other without worry. When the owner gets up, they follow 30 seconds later. And then watch out when the person turns around! Pear Buns will undoubtedly go in the opposite direction. To those who own them I can only say, "Bury the sugar bowl. Remember the Bunnetics curse and get to work!"

JELLY BUNS

(Medium to small, sort of soft, either sagging or starting to sag.) Without question, Jelly Buns are cute, "Like a baby's tusche," the saying goes. If you are young and good looking, you can get away with them. But even then, when "body mortis" (the thirtieth birthday) starts to set in, help better be on the way, or the distance between them and the back of your knees gets shorter and shorter. Fortunately, with regular and persistent work, they are the easiest to shape up.

PRESTO BUNS

(Flat and shapeless.) Remember Mandrake the Magician's "Now you see it, PRESTO! Now you don't"? If you turn your back to the mirror, Presto buns are there, but don't turn profile because you will see only the back wall. Look through the Bunnetic exercises and you will find plenty of help without having to wish for a pair of Magic Buns out of a top hat. Gaining a little weight will help, too. If all else fails and it means a lot to you, go see the Broadway musical *A Chorus Line*. One of the characters found the answer to your problem on New York's Park Avenue and 73rd Street.

DUNE BUNS

(Just perfect.) Dune Buns are tops, and their owners know it. Summer belongs to them! On the beach they compete with the environment, and win. You never see their owners' faces, but who cares? These dream buns are always clad in designer trunks with the label discretely on the side. They ride the best bicycles, never jog on side streets (only main thoroughfares), and like to wear old faded-out jeans with smartly torn holes and patches.

FLAMENCO BUNS

(As tough and snappy as castanets.) These are my favorite. Most dancers have them, but they can also be found in bull rings and Latin Fiestas. They are full of rhythm and pizazz, but their beauty is often shadowed by an arched back, pinned back shoulders, and weak stomach muscles. Bunnetic exercises can easily correct that, then, on with the show. La Cucaracha, la cucaracha . . .

So here you are, six different groupings to choose from. All of the Bunnetic exercises will be beneficial to any group. Even if you have Dune Buns, you want to keep them that way, don't you? Those exercises that I feel are essential to one specific group are indicated in the appropriate places. To start The Plan you will need a couple of minor accessories, and once you have them you are ready. They are:

1. A tape measure.
2. A soft blanket or rug you can lie on.
3. A pair of loose-fitting shorts or exercise pants.
4. A roll of plastic paper wrap (the type that adheres to containers), and a few rolls of it in storage.

The first three implements are self-explanatory. The fourth is necessary for the Bun Warmers. This easy-to-make contraption, used properly and regularly, will help you reduce inches from the lower stomach, hips, and buns. Wearing it creates insulated heat that takes water from the fat cells of your skin and consequently makes it easier for your body to eliminate fat. Contrary to popular opinion, fat cells, once you have them, do not go away. They get "skinnier" but do not disappear. That is why people who go on and off crash diets keep losing and gaining. Their fat cells (adipose cells) just take a vacation knowing that soon they are going to be filled again unless the individual shocks them by changing his or her eating habits. Only then do they go inert. In short, the Warmer helps get rid of water but does not burn the fat. Fat cells are filled with oil and water. Oil burns at 360 degrees, so only your restriction of calories is going to help burn that fat.

Dancers use a kind of loose sweat suit made up of a plastic or vinyl fabric that can be bought in dance-wear shops. It has the same effect as the Warmer, but I prefer the wrapping paper. The suit is too easy to wear for long periods, which is not advisable. If you do buy one, make sure you wear it *only* while doing the movements at home. Put it on 10 minutes before you start and take it off right after you finish. They are most effective when worn over wool or heavy knit pants. The Bun Warmer, in contrast, allows the air to circulate between the skin and the paper and so can be worn throughout the day under your clothes, but if you do so, it will have to be changed frequently. Here is how you make it.

THE BUN WARMER

1. Face the mirror if necessary.

2. Take the roll in the right hand[1] and the loose edge in the left, and roll out about 10 inches of it. Don't cut it!

3. Place the edge of the sheet in the center line of the body, with half of its width below the navel and the other half above it.

4. Holding the edge on this position, wrap over the right side of your body, around the lower back, over the left side to the front and over the starting line. Press and it will cling together.

5. Roll down to the back of the right thigh, around to the inside of the leg, and over to the front of the thigh.

6. Roll it over the right bun and the left bun and bring it over the left hip.

7. Take it down over the top of the left thigh, wrap it around the inside of the thigh, bring it out from behind to the front over the left side. Take it up to the starting point. Clip it and cling it. It's done.

---

[1] Since I am right-handed it is easier for me to hold the roll in the right hand. If you are left-handed, just reverse the instructions. I suggest you take a couple of practice shots so that when you start on Buns One you are wrapped up expertly.

Laying the Foundation— The Bottom Line

By now the Pre-Buns conditioners should have given your two bubbles a little burst of what's to come, and your mind should be ready for your new endeavor. You have read this far and your anxiety has built up. Did you reflexively grab for a chocolate bar during the first pages? How many jeans' commercials have you seen since you bought this book? Have all those perfect derrieres made you envious? I bet you told yourself you could never come close to looking half that good. Well, you can. It is going to take work, a word we don't often like, but we are going to make the work fun. FUN WITH BUNS! Corny, isn't it? Never mind. When you get through with this plan you'll see that corniness had hidden advantages.

All right—let's get to it. Pencil sharpened? Tape measure ready? It's going to hurt a little, but what the hell, YOU ARE DETERMINED. If you're not in front of a mirror, you'd better get to one. Quickly. There is no time to lose.

Ready? Take all your clothes off, and take a good look. Be truthful with yourself. Most of us are our own worst critics. No one I know is 100 percent pleased with his or her body. Just remember that no one is built the same. What you see in front of you is unique—there is not another one like it in the whole world. You are exclusive! Original! And all you are going to do is add some finishing touches to make you more beautiful. Now measure around the waist, right above the hip bones about 2 inches below the rib cage. That is where most pants fit. If you can't feel an indentation, do not get hysterical, you are just a little fatter than you think. If you have a broad frame, it might take a little poking around; but your waist is there.

Measure first by pulling the stomach in tight and pushing the chest out high. Make a note on the left side of the pad. Now let it all hang out and measure again. Dry those tears! Make a "truthful" note on the right side of the pad and divide the difference in the two measurements in half. Losing that many inches is your first goal.

Now the real toughy. Measure around the lower stomach. Make sure the tape rests right on the origin of your buns (The Top Line), just below the lower back. Again: Pull in tight, measure and write, then relax and measure. Let that four-letter word out if it makes you feel better, and then write.

To the center of the problem! Turn around and look at yourself in profile. If you have always thought one of your sides is better than the other, use that one first, but I guarantee you they are both going to be the same. Place the tape around the exact middle of your buns. Tightening won't make much of a difference here, especially if you are overly cushioned. So what you get is what you write, and don't cheat by tightening the tape either.

Next, to the right leg. Place the tape around the top of your leg, from the groin outward. Keep it horizontal to the floor. Tightening your leg here won't make much difference either, so just write down the first measurement. Then do the same with the left leg. There might be a slight difference. Don't worry, that's not uncommon.

Finally, place the tape on the line where your Buns end and the legs start (The Bottom Line). Bring it around both sides to the front. Keep it horizontal to the floor. Measure it. Tighten and measure again. Though there won't be much difference, write it down and divide. This is the most important area, since due both to the weight of the buns and the poor toning of them, it drops earliest and fastest on a person. This area also gives that sexy, round look.

Let's summarize what you should have written down:

	Tight	(Relax) Actual	Difference	Goal 2nd wk.	4th wk.	6th wk.
1. Waist measurement	X	X	X			
2. Lower stomach (*Top Line*)	X	X	X			
3. Buns (*Mid Line*)	X	X				

	(Relax) Tight	Actual	Difference	Goal 2nd wk.	4th wk.	6th wk.
4. Right leg (*top*)		X				
5. Left leg (*top*)		X				
6. Both legs (*Bottom Line*)	X	X	X			

You are on your way. Remember, you are going to repeat this procedure every two weeks for six weeks. The measurements at the end of the first two weeks will not be very exciting. But if you eat properly and do the exercises regularly, you'd better save your money for those new jeans because the measurements after the fourth week are going to freak you out.

More About Bunnetics

At this time I think it is important to state that my plan is not a complete shape-up plan. Such a plan to be effective should have some personal supervision and be tailored to the individual's physical state and need. But if you do minimal or no exercise at all, the Bunnetics plan will bring you closer to an ideal level of muscle firmness, strength, and coordination resulting in a loss of inches from localized areas. If you are a physically active person, you will find Bunnetics an excellent way to further develop stretch, flexibility, muscle tone, and firmness in areas—like the buns and stomach—that most sports do not work hard enough. However, the Bunnetics program, as it appears in this book, is not a cardiovascular endurance system, since the exercises are not long, fast, or repetitive enough for cardiovascular expansion. For the purpose of endurance and a stronger heart, I recommend aerobic exercises such as jogging, swimming, and aerobic dance—and the last only in places that specialize in aerobic dance, and not just as a part of other programs.

Although dancers seldom do it because it tightens leg muscles, jogging has become the most popular of all forms of aerobic exercise. As in all unsupervised exercise programs, jogging has its short-comings. Among them is that many people who go wild with it have developed kidney problems due to its bouncy action, and some gynecologists have been known to forbid it to patients be-cause of uterus-related problems. People with knee and lower back problems may also find jogging a little hazardous. Check with your doctor before you embark on a jogging spree.

Swimming is still the most complete of all forms of exercises, with the only deterrent being the need for lots of water nearby, not to mention a hair dryer. In New York City, at the 63rd Street Y.M.C.A.—located just a couple of blocks from Lincoln Center for the Performing Arts—it is not uncommon to see the Y's large pool being used by famous dancers. Many of them are swimming under doctor's advice in order to heal dance-related injuries. I love to swim but hate pools, and since *Jaws* I won't be caught dead in the ocean. If you are going to swim you don't have to be a Mark Spitz, but remember that the dog paddle will only recede your cuticles, not your buns.

Aerobic dance, an old fad now renewed by new tunes (the disco beat) is nothing more than dancing in a sweat shop. Obviously, I am partial to anything that has to do with dance, but when you go to a place that offers it, do not be afraid to ask who devised the program. It is also advisable to know the qualifications of that person, as well as that of the instructor or leader. Some places ask for a brief medical history and even a basic examination as well as a waver of liability. Such care is not without reason. Too much energy often results in bad skeletal alignment, back pains, dizziness, and pulled or sore muscles. Beware! The best places have a graded program.

The key to exercising is patience. You must start with moderation and build up speed or intensity as you progress. It is the quality, the rhythm, and the continuity of what you do that will give you results, not the strength alone. Force usually discourages you and can be a cause for forgetting all your good intentions. Use the Bunnetic exercises and follow their escalation from Buns One to Buns Forever. I have tried to make them fun and easy. I hope you enjoy them. I know you will enjoy the results.

Let's get to work.

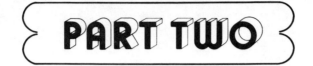

The Plan

This plan has shown great results with the average person after five weeks' time. I have chosen these exercises from the ones most favored for their results and ease of execution by students of my Bunnetic classes in New York City. If you are overweight and are not willing to do something about it, you are still welcome to follow my suggestions, but do not expect any miracles. If you have to lose over twenty pounds and have decided to go on a weight-reducing plan during Bunnetics, or you are already on one, some of the exercises will be hard to do at first. In this case do Buns One and Buns Two for an extra week each, and cut in half the amount of time suggested for the exercises for the first week. Do the second week in full, and continue The Plan as suggested. I am aware that the majority of people do not follow orders to the letter. In the forming of Bunnetics I have taken that into consideration, but the fact remains that the closer you follow The Plan, the better the results will be.

The Plan should be done twice a day, the first time in the morning before a full breakfast. (You can have the morning coffee. Nothing should ever be done before that, except perhaps crawling out of bed and switching on the bathroom light. So have the coffee, and take the dog out. You can put on your Bun Warmer while the coffee is brewing and have it on while walking Spot.)

Then you should repeat The Plan again in the evening. Bunnetic movements are designed to alleviate the tension gathered after a long, tiring day, as well as working the parts of the body most neglected during the day. Ideally, they should be done before dinner, but if this is not possible, then you should wait two hours after eating. They also are a great preparation for a good night's sleep. You just can't skip doing The Plan at night, unless you substitute with "For Couples Only." These exercises are the most fun and full of surprises.

The Plan is divided into four weeks of conditioning exercises. Each week certain movements are added, intensified, and then changed. Thus, Buns One will be easier than Buns Two, and Two, easier than Buns Three, etc. Each segment has a Warm-up Period that remains the same throughout. The progression of the exercises through the first four weeks all lead to the exercises of the fifth week, Buns Forever. After completing your fifth week, the object is for you to continue shaping, reducing, and staying fit through the Buns Forever sequence by doing it a minimum of twice a week.

A problem that I know many of you will encounter is that exercising alone isn't as much fun as with someone else or a group of people. Dancers will sweat up a storm in class without hesitation, but very few will actually stretch at home. The right environment must be created for psychological motivation. I wouldn't recommend you hang out the window and invite a passerby to come up and exercise, but I am sure that you could invite a few friends for a Bunnetic dinner party and then challenge a couple of them to reduce right along with you. (Before you set the plates down, of course.)

Don't worry about how long it is going to take you to get your body where you want it. The fact that you have decided to do something about it and embarked on it is in itself harder to do than any of the exercises will be. When doing the exercises, take the time to read the instructions, understand them, and assimilate them. Pay attention to the Starting Positions and their instructions on posture and alignment. They will help you to do the exercises with much more ease and without unnecessary output of energy.

You do not have to feel rivers of perspiration to know you are exercising. Most of the exercises are designed to be done at a slow to medium pace. You should know that the slower you do the movements, the harder it is to do them, and the longer it may take you to do them well. But their benefits will stay with you longer, too.

Here are some additional suggestions that will help you with The Plan:

1. Select a place to do Bunnetics and make it your own private gym.

2. Have a couple of outfits that you can wear exclusively for this purpose. Once you put them on you will feel more like starting.

3. Music can be very stimulating, but not classical music. If you

have a record player, get some disco or disco-fused jazz records. Ask the salesperson for medium-dance-tempo ones.

4. If one particular day you just don't feel well or don't feel like exercising, don't force yourself. Do just the Warm-ups.

5. For those of you with Presto Buns, Jelly Buns, or excessive cellulite, a set of 3–5-pound ankle weights, available at most sporting goods stores, can be of great help in the exercises where their use is indicated. Check with a doctor before trying them.

The Warm-up

Although there are some physiologists who have reported that a warm-up period is neither beneficial nor harmful, there are thousands of dancers and athletes who would tell these people that they are plain crazy. A warm-up period before any kind of out-of-the-ordinary physical activity is a must for increasing the oxygen and blood supply to the muscle fibers, thus allowing better contractile action with less use of energy. This is true especially when exercises are done in the morning, after the body has received a long rest and has functioned at minimal energy consumption. The most common result of skipping a warm-up is cramps, which are caused by insufficient blood supply to the muscle.

The following Warm-ups are designed to increase the blood supply to the various muscles that work during the exercises; to create a balanced skeletal position; to activate your thinking process during the movements through the use of imagery (neuromuscular activity); and to prepare the body for the Bunnetic Plans.

The RP (Rest Position)

Before starting the Warm-up movements you must align your body through the use of this very restful position. Sit on the floor and bend your knees with the feet flat on the floor and as close to the pelvis as possible. Place both hands on your hips with your thumbs toward your back and fingers pointing toward the groin area. Rock slightly from side to side and you will feel little bulging movements under your fingers. That is the hip joint, where the leg bone (the femur) connects with the hip. Make sure that each knee is in a straight line up and away from each joint, and each foot is in direct line downward from its corresponding knee. This should form a 90° angle in each leg (a triangle from the floor). Both legs should run parallel to one another, their separation equal to the distance between both hip joints.

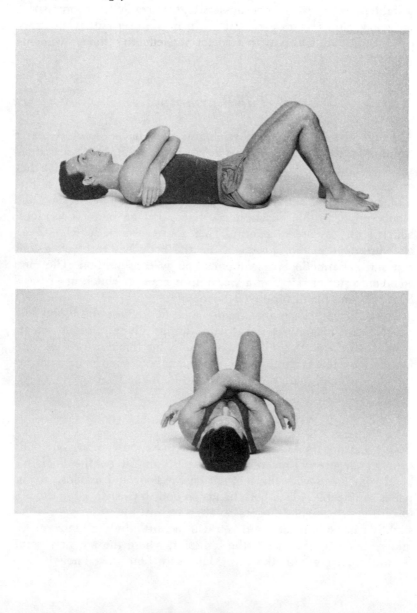

Now lie back and cross the arms over the chest as indicated. This will help to extend the shoulder blades and to flatten the back against the floor. If your upper back muscles are tense, they will tend to pull the arms down, making it difficult to keep your arms in this position. Soon it will become easier. Give yourself a couple of minutes' rest in this position, breathing as evenly as possible. It helps to imagine yourself floating in a nice warm bath. The more rested the body is, the more efficient and effective the movements will be because there won't be interference from muscles that could tighten up. All Warm-ups start in the RP; you are ready for the first one.

The Bridge

(*Image:* You are a draw bridge over a wide river. Your Pelvis is the fixed point of the bridge. Your torso is the lift-up platform, and your head is its end. Water is flowing right under your back.)

1. Concentrate on lifting up this bridge as much as you can while maintaining a straight back. Your goal is to eventually reach a 45° angle from the floor. If you can do it now, you are in better shape than you think. Count to ten while doing this.[1]

2. When you're lifted as close to 45° as you can get, contract your stomach as hard as you can and hold the position for 10 counts. Bring the bridge down slowly to rest, counting backward from 10.

3. Lie and rest for 10 counts.

4. Then, still lying down, contract the stomach again for another 10 counts.

5. Rest for 10 counts.

---

[1] All counting must be done aloud for proper breathing. The breath should never be held, even in the strongest of contractions.

The Sponge

(*Image:* Think of your buns as a huge sponge saturated with water. This might be closer to reality than you think.)

1. As if you were squeezing the water in the sponge with your fingers, do 10 very light and fast contractions with your buns. This will be felt primarily on the sphyncter muscle, deep inside the rectum.

2. Now squeeze the sponge as hard as you can and hold for 10 counts.

3. Relax for 10 counts.

4. Repeat 3 times for a total of 4.

The Oyster

Still in the RP, bring your thighs together so that their insides touch, as well as the inside edges of your feet. Depending on the skeletal structure of your legs, the act of bringing your feet together will range from easy to impossible. The most important thing is that the inside of your thighs are touching and your feet are flat on the floor.

(*Image:* Your legs are now an oyster deep on the bottom of the ocean surrounded by thousands of pounds of water pressure that help to seal it shut.)

1. Tighten your buns while pressing the thighs together for 10 counts. Release and relax for 10 counts.

2. Take 10 counts to open the legs as wide as possible, trying to keep the heels and toes of the feet together, and imagining the strong water pressure that is fighting your opening them.

3. When you reach maximum opening, contract your buns for 10 counts.

4. Relax and slowly close the legs again.

5. Repeat.

The Glass Dropper

Start with your legs in open position with the bottom of the feet together (as the end of Step 2 of **The Oyster**).

(*Image:* You are a water-filled glass dropper, with your buns the rubber cap which when squeezed presses the water down the glass tube formed by your legs. Your feet are the orifice out of which the water drips.)

1. Squeeze your buns and at the same time slide the legs down, with the heels on the floor until the feet open out and the legs straighten. 10 counts.

2. Release the squeeze and bring the legs to the starting position. 10 counts.

3. Repeat 3 more times for a total of 4.

You have finished your Warm-up and are ready for the Buns Plan. Remember that the first time everything will take you a little longer to do. Practice makes perfect (and it makes the exercises go faster, too).

Buns One

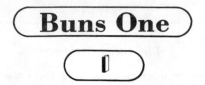

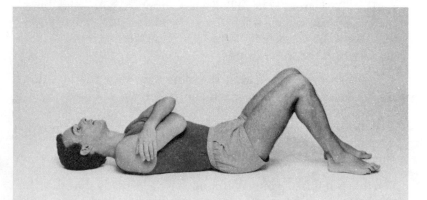

Starting Position: The RP.
Squeeze buns as tight as possible for 8 counts, then relax for another 8 counts. Though you can't see it, I really *am* squeezing.

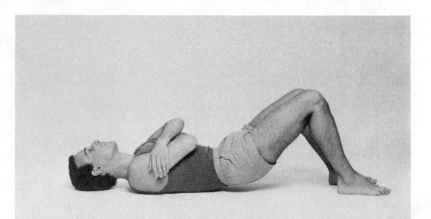

Lift pelvis up off the floor and place it down. Squeeze tight when going up; relax when going down. Do it twice. Make sure that your lower back stays resting on the floor.

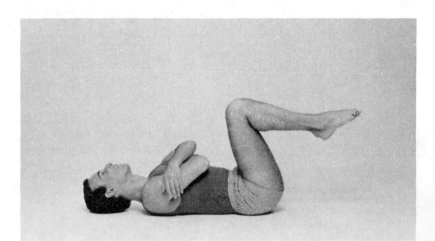

Keeping buns on the floor and knees apart but parallel, lift knees toward the chest then lower them until feet touch the floor. Do this twice.

Now repeat the entire set.

Here Biggie and Tiny battle Mini.

Starting Position: Arms in RP, but legs extended and resting on the floor.

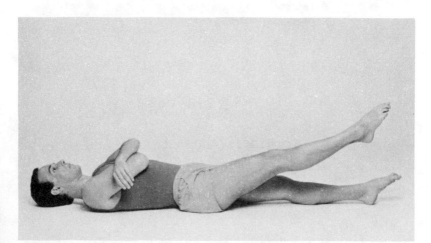

Lift leg (no more than 40°) and tighten buns and leg muscles for 8 counts. Relax the leg muscle but continue to hold the leg up for another 8 counts.

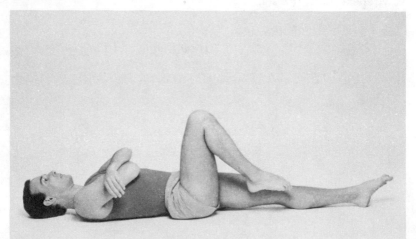

With the leg still off the floor, bend the knee and bring the foot close to the pelvis and in line with hip joint.

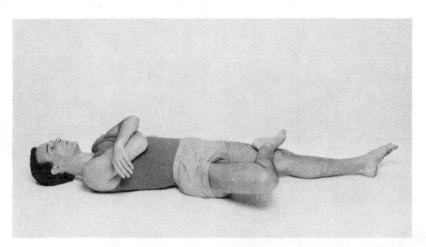

Rotate the leg to the side, lowering the knee close to floor and resting the foot over the extended thigh. Bring it back up and then extend the leg. Let it rest on the floor, then immediately do the same movements with the other leg.

Repeat entire set on both sides.

Even the hardest Flamenco Buns need their Sartorii worked.

Starting Position: With legs extended on the floor, rest arms along-side the body. Pull in the stomach tightly while pressing arms hard against the floor. Hold for 8 counts and relax for 8 counts. Then:

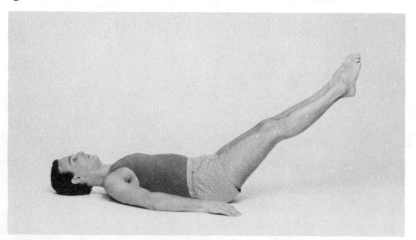

Lift both legs as slowly as possible (just 45°). When lifting the legs you must try to keep the stomach relaxed. This is easier if you continue a light press on the floor with the arms. Big Buns, Mini, and Quads get a jolt out of this one!

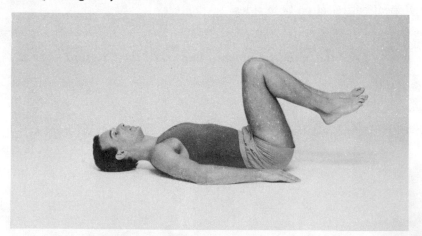

Bend your knees but keep the back flat against the floor.

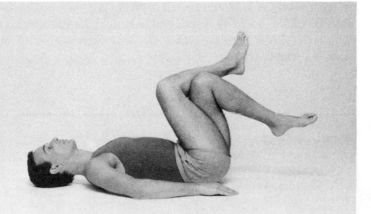

Now cross right thigh over left. Bring them back to parallel position, then place both feet on the floor and slide them down until
reaching starting position. Repeat, this time crossing left over right.
Do one slow set and one fast one.

*Pear, Bumper, and Jelly Buns do one extra set.
Remember the curse!*

Starting Position: Lie on your left side with both knees together and bent toward chest, as in a fetal position. Thighs should form a 90° angle with trunk, and back should be flat not curved. Elbows are together with head resting on hands. This will help to keep neck and spine in a straighter alignment. A small pillow between hands and head could be used, but not in the early morning. You might never make it to the office. In this exercise Tessie and the Quads will yell for help.

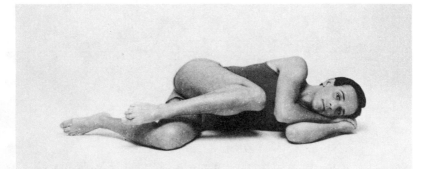

Bring right knee to chest. Swing it back past the left knee in an upward curve, keeping both the knee and the leg facing straight ahead, and maintaining the bent knee.

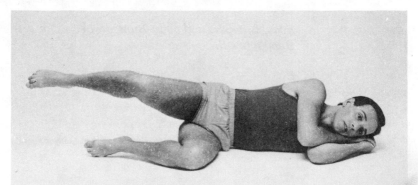

Do 2 very slow sets (4 counts up and 4 counts out). Then do for 8 fast counts (1 count up and 1 count out).

Buns of the World, Awake!

Starting Position: Try to assume the position indicated below, and then carefully read the following instructions.

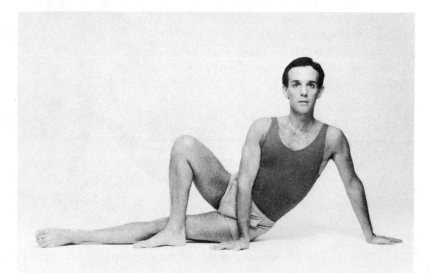

Place your left hand on the floor with the fingers pointing away from the body. Place the right arm in a straight line down from the right shoulder. Lean the torso against the arms, as you keep the left side of the torso stretched and the shoulders down. Keep the right knee bent with the foot directly in front of the left knee, and the toes pointing to the right.

As you execute the exercise you must concentrate on keeping the bent knee in line with the body and not allowing it to tilt forward. The torso must also be as erect as possible throughout. This exercise is one of the hardest you will find, but extremely beneficial to hip line, torso, and inner thigh.

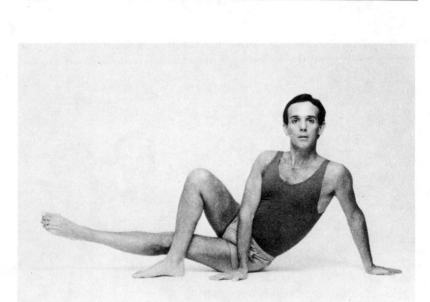

Now lift the left leg off the floor and hold for 8 counts.

Relax and repeat. If you find this impossible, then slide the right foot farther down the left leg and try it again, but having the right foot in front of the left knee is the object.

This exercise is a must for toning the Adductor group, Tessie and Tiny.

Dune Buns repeat twice.

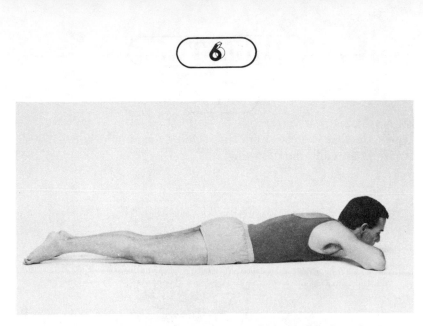

Starting Position: Lie face down with legs extended. Lift up one leg, keeping the hip bone on the floor.

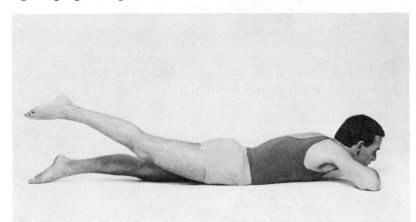

Hold it up and tighten buns and thigh for 8 counts. Relax before placing it on the floor again. Do the same with the other leg, then alternate lifting and placing each leg 8 times quickly.

(The use of ankle weights does wonders for Presto, Dune, and Jelly Buns in this exercise.)

Presto Buns: 3 extra sets.

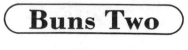

Buns Two

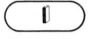

Repeat the first exercise from Buns One (you should know it well by now), then add the following:

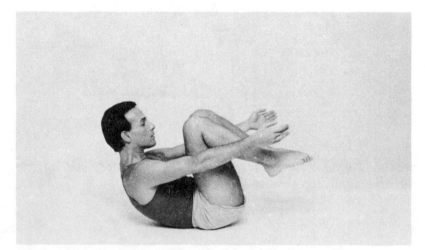

Bring the knees toward the chest while lifting the torso 45° off the floor. The arms reach around the legs.

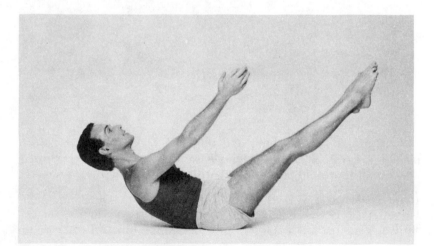

Extend legs and arms upward.

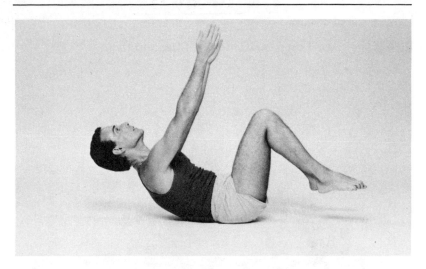

Bend the knees while keeping the torso off the floor. The arms reach up to the ceiling.

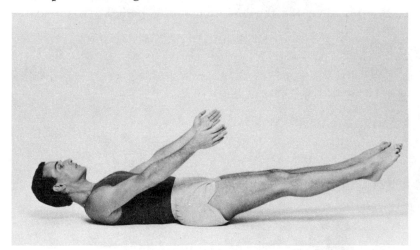

Extend the legs without placing them on floor. Rest the torso on the floor but continue to reach out with the arms. Repeat one more time.

This exercise is no fun, but you can practically see your stomach harden, your back strengthen, and your buns firm up after each time.

Repeat the second exercise from Buns One, and then:

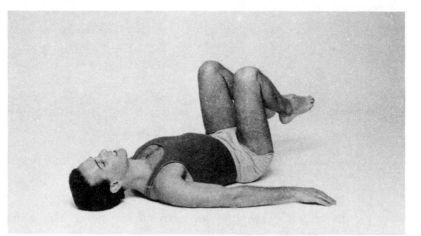

Place arms alongside the body and bring both knees up to the chest.

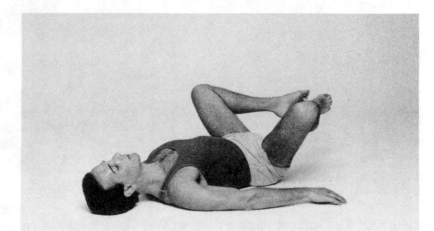

Press the knees outward, keeping the bottoms of the feet facing each other, but not together. Close the legs again and then extend them down the floor, but don't rest them.

Repeat 3 times.

Repeat the third exercise from Buns One, then add the following:

Starting Position: Lift both legs up to a 45° angle from the floor. Bend your knees, remembering to always keep them apart and parallel. Then:

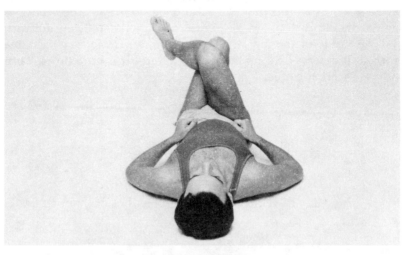

Cross right over left. Switch and cross left over right. Continue to alternate crossings for a total of 16 times (8 each leg).

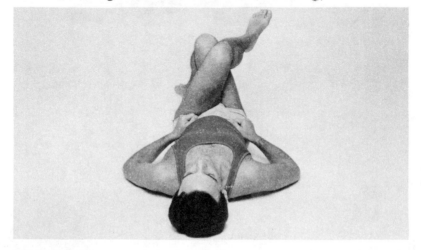

This one gives everybody a good workout and it is great for Thunder Thighs!

Repeat the fourth exercise from Buns One, then add the following:

Continue to bring the knee up to the chest, but now straighten it as you swing it back out, keeping the inside of the thigh a few inches off the floor. From this position, lift the leg up toward the ceiling as high as the hip will allow. You must keep the knee facing forward and the inside of the leg facing the floor, or Tessie won't get the workout it deserves. Swing the leg back and lift it up 8 times. Turn over and work the other leg.

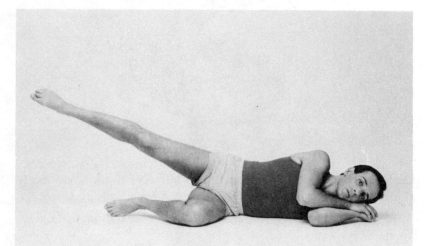

Repeat the fifth exercise from Buns One, and then add the following:

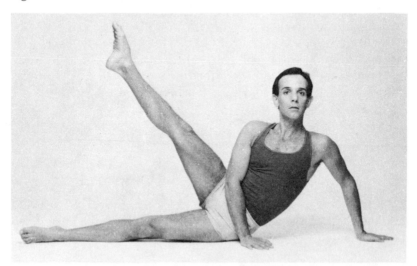

Extend the bent leg until the knee straightens. Keep the foot pointed, then return to starting position.

Now lift the inside leg up and place it down. Do it slowly. Then follow this lift with an extension. Continue alternations for a total of 8 times each.

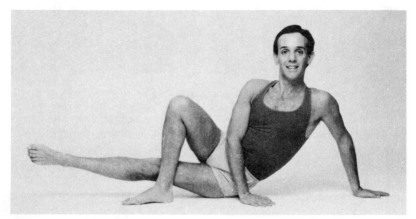

Flamenco Buns Olé for 8 more.

Repeat the sixth exercise from Buns One, then add the following:

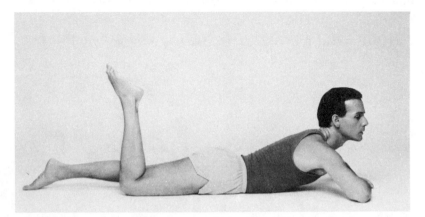

Push the chest off the floor and bend the right leg at the knee. Keep the toes pointed.

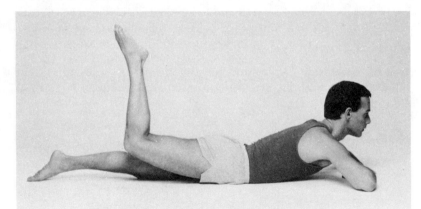

With buns relaxed, lower leg straightened, and both hip bones on the floor, lift the right thigh up and place it down. Progressively work to a minimum of 8 lifts. Rest a moment, then do the left leg. This really works the hamstrings, which tend to cramp when they have had enough.

Pear and Presto Buns can't skip this one.

Floor Stretch

Starting Position: Lie on the floor face down, elbows out and at shoulder level. Your legs should be straight and in line with the hip bones.

Take a few seconds to relax in this position, then slowly:

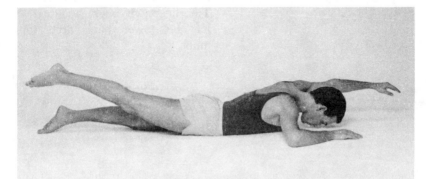

Lift the right leg while extending the left arm forward along the side of the head. Try to reach as far forward with the arm, and as far back with the leg, as possible. Place the leg down and bring arm in. Do the same with the other leg and arm. Take your time. If you feel tense, a couple of more times will help to relax you. Finish by lifting both arms over the head and both legs off the floor.

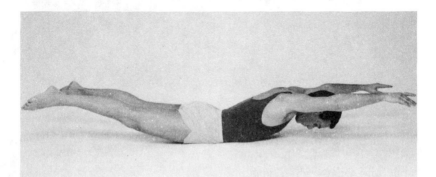

Both the pelvis and the stomach must stay on the floor. Do the movements slowly, stretching out, breathing evenly, and holding each position for a few seconds.

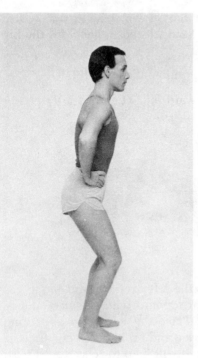

Starting Position: Stand up with the feet slightly apart (hip-joint width) and the knees bent. Place hands on hips and incline the upper torso forward. Then: Tilt the pelvis back, but do not let the lower back arch too much.

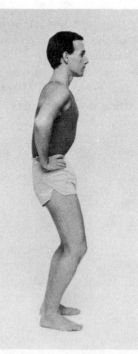

Now push the pelvis forward and up. Tighten the Buns, Hams, and Quads when pushing forward, and relax them when tilting back. Continue this back-front motion for 24 counts.

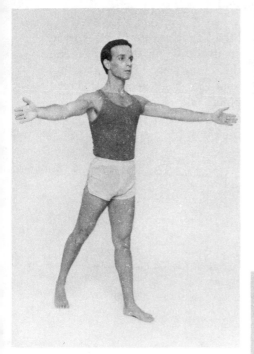

Starting Position: Stand on one leg with the other leg extended back and only its toes on the floor. This will help you keep your weight mostly on the forward leg. The arms are open to the side.

Reach forward with the arms as you bend your standing leg, while bringing the back leg forward, knee toward chest. Return to starting position. Try 16 counts on each side.

NOTE: Bad balance and poor posture are a result of weak muscle tone and/or poor skeletal alignment. Standing on one leg may be hard at first. Persevere and you will soon feel the difference. The arm movement helps to firm the Lats.

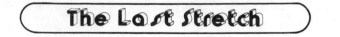

The Last Stretch

You will find this a fabulous way to end all our sequences.

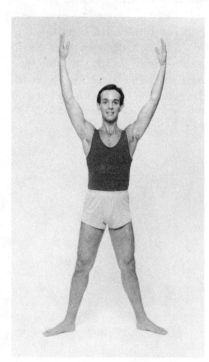

Stand with your legs spread comfortably apart and rotate them outward from the hip joint so that feet and knees point out. Keep the arms up and shoulders down. Tighten the buns.

Keeping the weight centered between both legs, incline the body forward as the knees bend. Keep reaching forward with arms to keep the back straight and elongated. As you get lower, your knees should be directly over your feet.

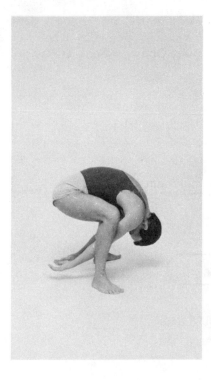

Lower the chin to the chest, and with the arms between the legs, reach toward the back wall until you round into an egg-like shape.

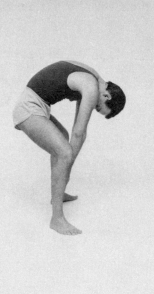

Slowly straighten. Pull in your stomach and continue to tighten it as you unfold slowly upward until you reach the starting position.

Repeat at least once.

Now get your measuring tape and stay away from the chocolate cookies!

Buns Three

Though at first glance this looks like a restful week, you'll think otherwise once you realize that this crucial period is when you intensify the work you learned in Buns One and Buns Two. April Fools!

Do the first exercise in Buns Two a minimum of 6 times.

Do Buns Two, No. 2, a minimum of 8 times.

Do the Buns Two, No. 3, and continue the thigh crossings for a minimum of 24 times (12 each leg).

Do Buns Two, No. 4, and continue the leg swing-and-lift for a minimum of 32 counts on each leg.

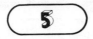

Do Buns Two, No. 5, then make it even harder by keeping the straight leg a few inches off the floor as you extend the bent leg toward the ceiling. Do 8 extensions, then rest before repeating on the other side.

Do Buns Two, No. 6. Then, after a very short pause, repeat it keeping the foot of the working leg flexed.

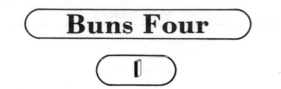

Buns Four

1

Starting Position: Keep the bottoms of the feet together and the knees out to the side. Place hands on the ankles and use them as an anchor to keep the torso lifted, spine erect and back flat.

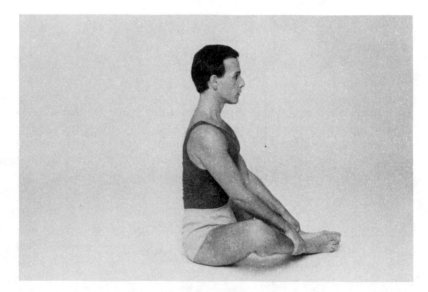

Contract and release the buns for 16 counts.

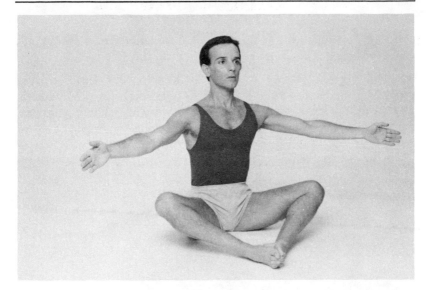

Now, concentrating on keeping back straight, chest up, and stomach pulled in, release the ankle hold and try to maintain erect posture (for at least 10 seconds) with arms open to the side.

NOTE: When the ankle hold is released the back will tend to collapse or curve. Don't let it. This isometric and isotonic exercise will strengthen the back, side, and stomach muscles and help to improve bad posture.

All Bunners with an arched back will benefit from this.

Starting Position: Sitting up straight, press the feet together and open the knees. The arms are straight out to the side.

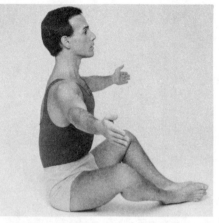

Keeping the knees pressed out, reach forward with the arms while slowly lying back on floor.

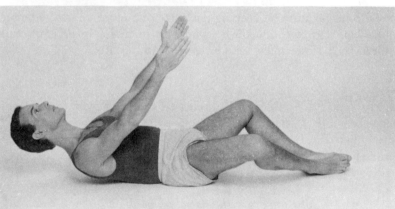

Slowly open the arms to the side as you sit up again. Try it 2 times slowly and then a minimum of 4 times faster.

This is a hard one, but Mini and Ester love it. You must try to keep knees from coming together when sitting up. That's the trick that makes this effective.

> *Pear Buns: 2 slow and 6 fast. Jelly, Presto, and Dune Buns: 4 slow and 8 fast.*

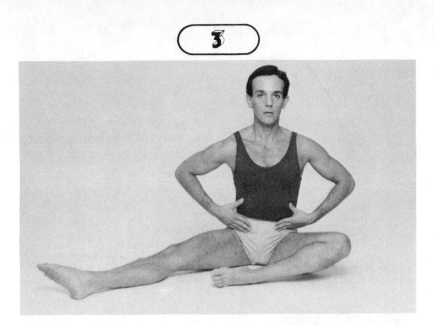

Starting Position: Keep the back straight and the right leg extended to the side. Bend the left knee and bring left foot in close to pelvis. Place hands on the waist, with elbows to the side but in line with chest.

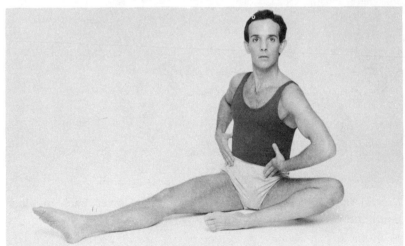

Keep looking straight ahead while twisting the torso from left to right for a minimum of 24 times (12 to each side). Those of you with sad Love Handles will feel them break into a smile. Change leg positions and repeat.

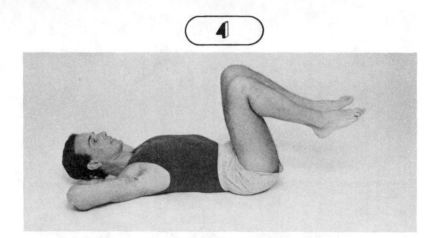

Lie on your back, and raise both knees, keeping them a few inches apart and parallel.

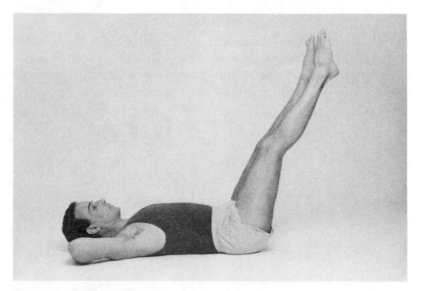

Extend the legs, and be sure to keep your lower back on floor. Bend and extend again.

Continue for a total of 16 counts, unless you pigged-out last night —then you should go for another 8.

Buns, the curse is still on!

Starting Position: Lie on your right hip, with legs together and in a straight line down from the torso. Keep the torso propped up through the support of the arms.

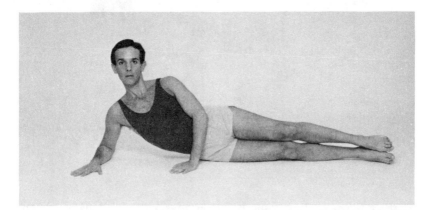

Bring the left knee toward chest at hip level. From this position, extend the leg straight ahead, then bend again and extend it down to the starting position. Repeat this process 8 times, then work the other side.

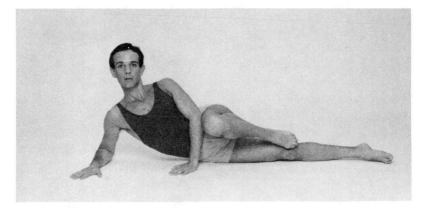

Keeping the torso propped up works the Lats and the Quads, while extending with the leg works the Buns.

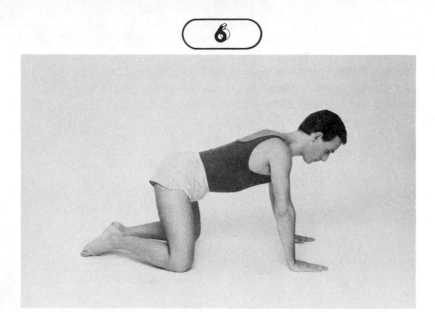

Starting Position: Rest your body on your knees and hands, keeping the feet together and the knees out. Keep the back straight and the fingers pointing forward and in direct line with knees. The elbows are slightly bent.

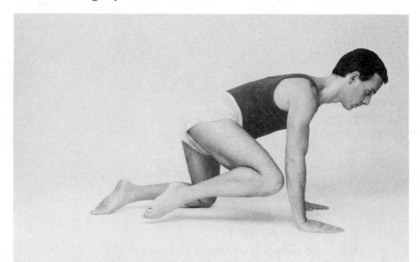

Lift the right knee and bring it forward to the right elbow. Avoid rolling to left side by letting your arms bear most of your weight.

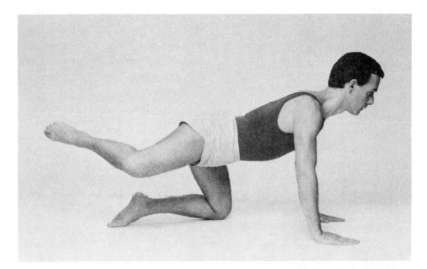

Swing the right leg back and up, keeping it bent and rotated out from hip joint. Bring it forward and swing it back 24 times, then work the other side. This is my Buns Food Processor. It blends, chops, and grinds away.

After completion do another Floor Stretch (page 67) before beginning the start of the next exercises.

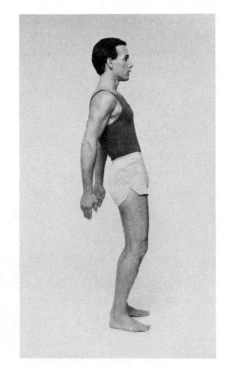

Starting Position: Start with feet parallel and the knees slightly bent. The pelvis is forward and the arms are slightly in back of the body.

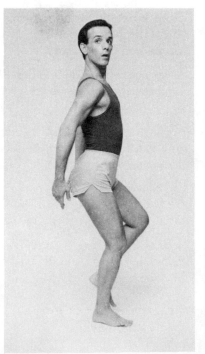

Lift the left knee off the floor and simultaneously tilt the pelvis back.

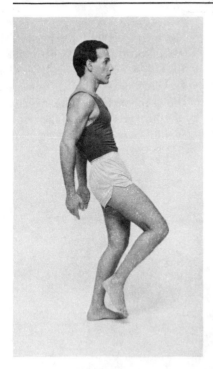

Step back on the left foot and at the same time pick up the right knee while tilting the pelvis forward. Keep the stomach pulled in.

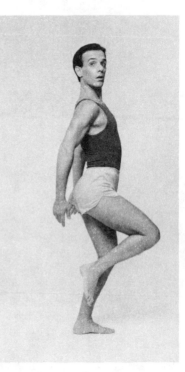

Bring the right knee farther up and at the same time tilt pelvis back.

Continue to walk back, coordinating the front and back motion of the pelvis with the steps. Walk back for 8 counts, then without altering the motion, walk forward for 8 counts.

NOTE: This requires a lot of slow-motion practice before you're able to develop a fast, coordinated walk without losing the continuity of the pelvic motion. It will not only work your thighs, lower abdomen, and lower back, but it might help you make it through the preliminaries if you ever audition for director-choreographer Bob Fosse. Persevere!

Flamenco and Dune Buns, here is where you can show off!

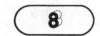

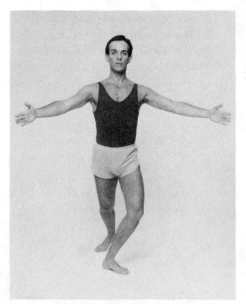

Starting Position: Keep the forward standing leg bent and the back leg extended. Notice that the legs are rotated out from the hip joint and the arms are to the side. Keep the body's weight over the front leg.

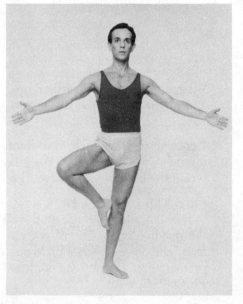

Bring the back leg forward with a bent knee to touch the inside of the standing knee, which should straighten as the back leg is lifted forward. Be sure to keep the bent leg rotated out.

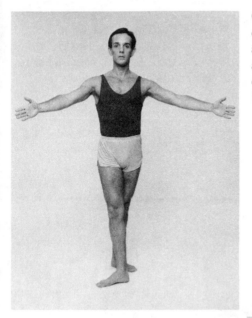

Cross the working leg in front of the standing leg and place it about 2 feet from it. Lift it up again, touching it to the inside of the other knee and place it back in the starting position.

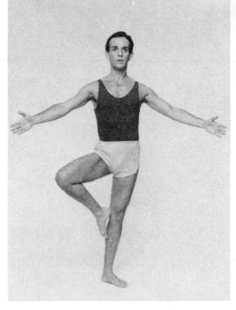

Continue for 16 counts, then work the other leg.

Buns work more when legs are rotated outward from the hip. Why else do you think ducks and ballet dancers have such nice ones?

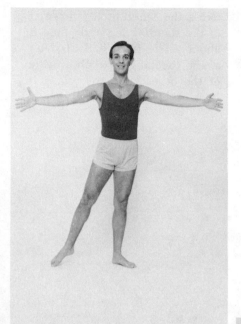

Starting Position: Start with the weight on the left leg, and right foot pointed to the side. The arms are opened out to the side.

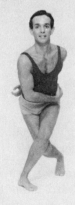

Cross the right thigh behind the left in a semi-bent position, and wrap the right arm around front of body and left arm around the back.

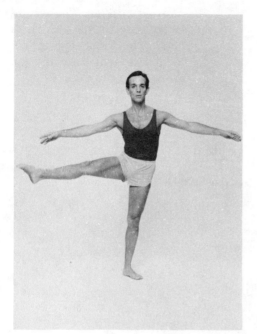

In one upward motion, swing the back leg to the side and open the arms. Return to the wrap position, then in one motion, come up, step to the right, and point the left foot to the left. You are now ready to work on the other side.

The faster you do this one the better. It works on all the muscle groups and it is an excellent aerobic movement. Try a minimum of 8 on each side.

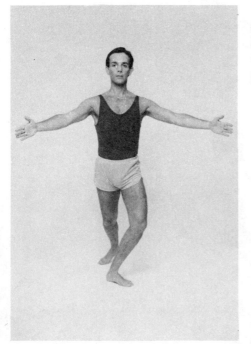

Starting Position: The weight is on the left leg, which is bent. The right leg is extended straight back and the arms are to the side.

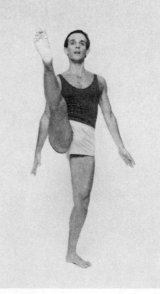

Kick the leg as high up as you can, and bring the arms down during the leg's upward swing. Return to the starting position. Try a minimum of 8 kicks with each leg.

This completes Buns Four. End with the Cooling-Down Stretch, and run for the measuring tape.

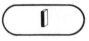

Dune Buns, fantasize and compare. Here's Darlene.

Repeat Buns Four, No. 1, then add the following:

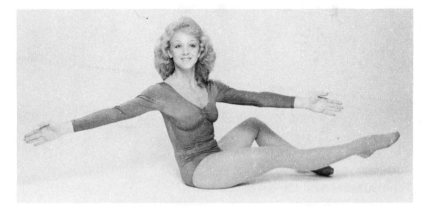

Twist the torso to the right and at the same time extend the right leg straight forward.

Face front again, folding in leg and arms. Repeat on the other side. Continue for 8 twists and extensions.

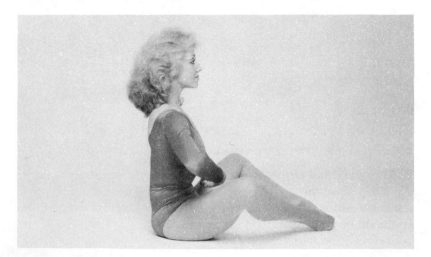

Repeat Buns Four, No. 2, then add the following:

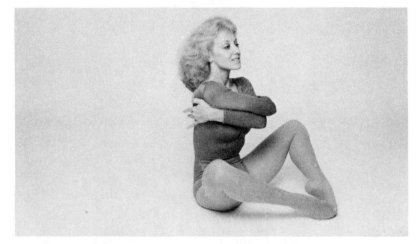

Wrap arms around the top of the body.

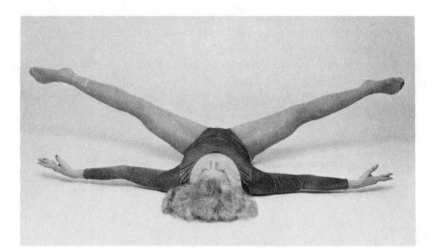

Now lie back and at the same time extend both legs straight out to the side. The arms go straight out as well. Then sit back up in starting position. Repeat this movement a minimum of 8 times, but 16 should be your goal.

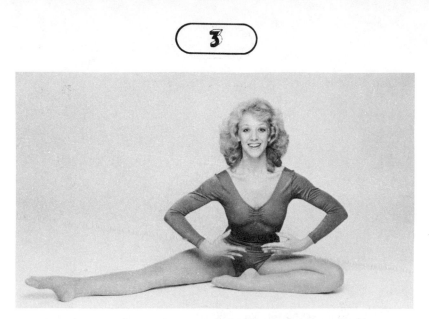

Do Buns Four, No. 3, right side only, 32 times. You'll finish in this position.

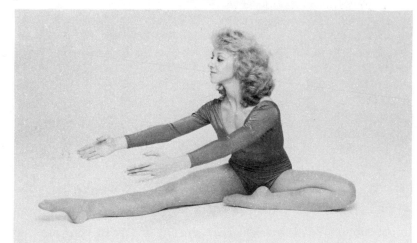

Now extend the arms over the extended leg. Keeping the stomach pulled in and the back straight, lean over to the extended foot. Then stretch toward the foot and pull back to upright position for a minimum of 8 times. Change leg positions, do Buns Four, No. 3, left side, 32 times, and repeat the above.

Biggie, Tiny, and Ester are asking the Hams to a party!

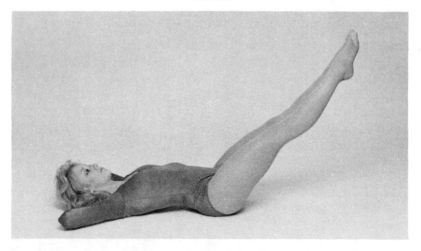

Repeat Buns Four, No. 4. You'll finish in this position, with the legs 45° off the floor and the hands laced together behind the head.

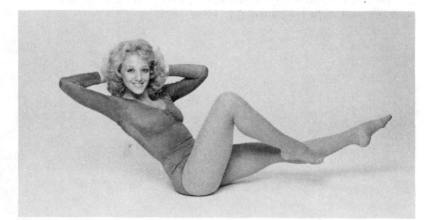

In one motion, bend the right knee and lift and twist your torso so that the left elbow reaches toward the right knee. Keep the left leg extended off the floor. Then twist the torso to the left, straightening the right leg and bending the left. Continue this motion of twisting and bending knees 6 times. Then lie back. Relax a second and repeat.

Ankle weights could be very beneficial in this exercise, especially for flabby stomachs and Jelly Buns.

Repeat Buns Four, No. 5, then add the following:

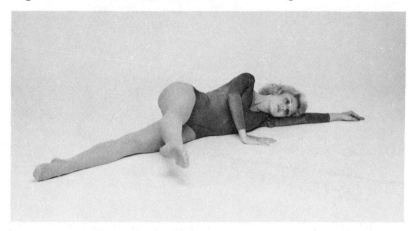

Now you are on your left hip. Rest your head on your extended arm and place the right hand on the floor to keep the torso from rolling back. Extend right leg forward to knee level.

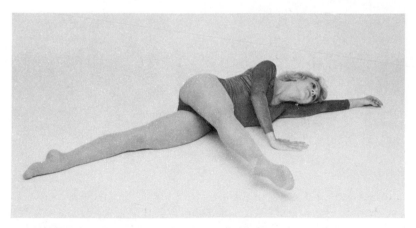

Push the leg up to hip level, and then back down to knee level. The movement is a pulsing one; do it 16 times. Roll over and do the other side.

If you use ankle weights on this one, cut the suggested repetitions in half or your buns and hamstrings will let you have it for a couple of days.

Repeat Buns Four, No. 6, and then add the following:

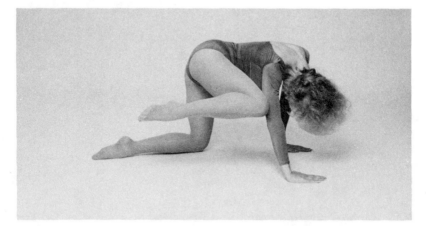

Touch the right knee to the right elbow. The head is down.

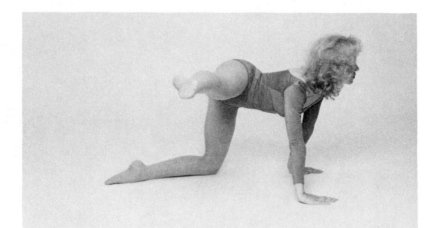

Extend the leg to the side, lifting the head and keeping the back straight. Then bring it back in to touch the elbow as you lower your head.

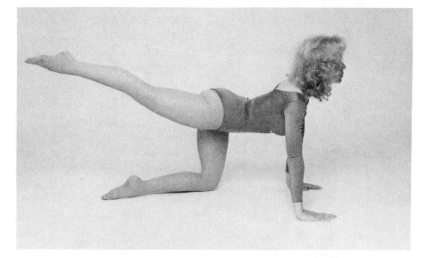

Extend the leg straight back, with the knee facing the floor. The head is lifted once again.

Repeat this sequence a minimum of 6 times on each side.

Follow up with the Floor Stretch.

Repeat Buns Four, No. 7, and then add the following:

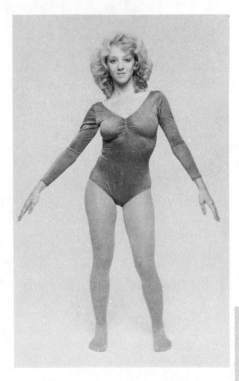

Start with weight centered evenly. The knees are bent, the feet are parallel, and the arms are to the side. Now lean your weight into the right hip.

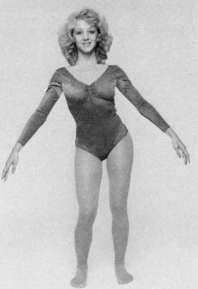

Now, to the left. Bump away 24 times.

A disco beat or riding a packed subway train can make this one energizing and very friendly.

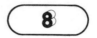

Repeat Buns Four, No. 8, and then add the following:

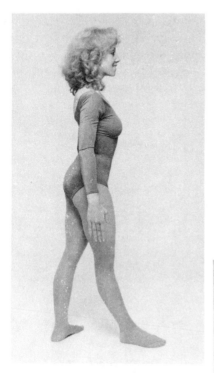

Place one leg in front of the other. Make sure to keep them rotated out from the hip joint. The arms are down and to the side.

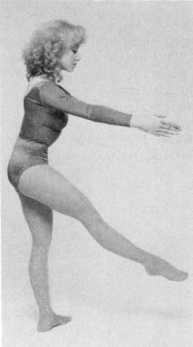

Lift the front leg up. As you bring the arms forward, lean forward slightly in the torso. Place the leg down and repeat for a total of 8 times on each leg.

Repeat Buns Four, No. 9, and then add the following:

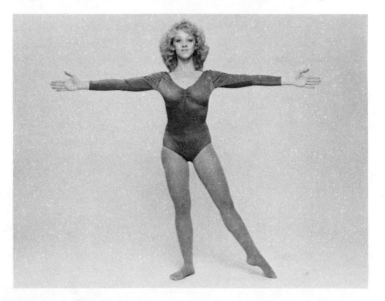

Stand on the right leg. Point the left leg to the side and open your arms straight out. Cross the left thigh behind the right one, and wrap the arms, left arm in front of the body, right arm behind. Try to get a little lower than last week in Buns Four.

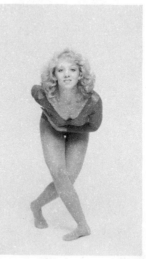

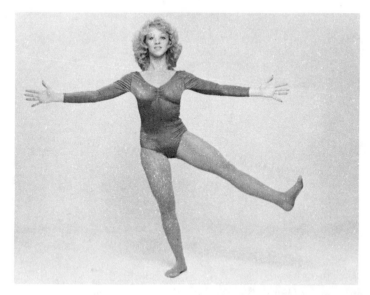

Come straight up again and kick the left leg to the side with the foot flexed. Bend and wrap, and straighten and kick, for a minimum of 12 kicks on each side.

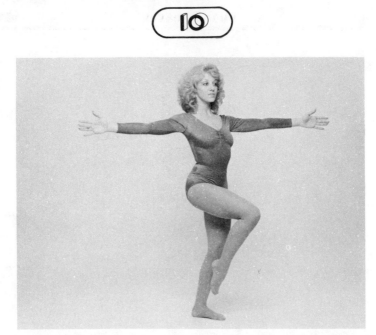

Repeat Buns Four, No. 10. After completing your full set of straight kicks, bend the working leg and extend it across body's midline. Make sure not to move the torso in the direction of extended leg; you should be twisted *against* the extension.

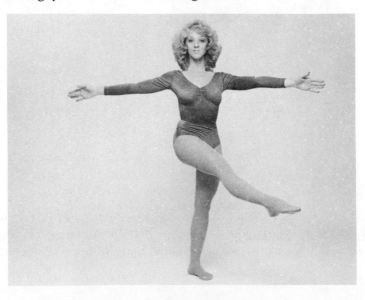

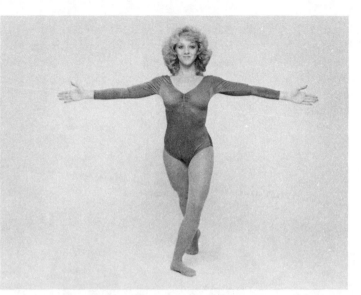

Bend the knee again and return to starting position. Do a minimum of 8 cross kicks on each side. The opposition movement of these cross kicks helps to trim Ester, the lower stomach, and the hip lines. The extension activates the buns.

Finish with the Cooling-Down Stretch.

By the end of this week you and your buns will be in better shape than ever. By continuing Buns Forever for a minimum of twice a week, you'll be able to keep your Dune Buns in shape all year long.

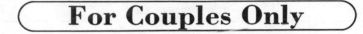

For Couples Only

Although at first glance the exercises of For Couples Only will seem like fun, and they are, their rewards are innumerable. But I must remind you that they are a supplement to the Bunnetics Plan and their effectiveness, as in the case of those in The Plan, depends entirely on the continuity of their use.

Have fun, you two!

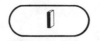

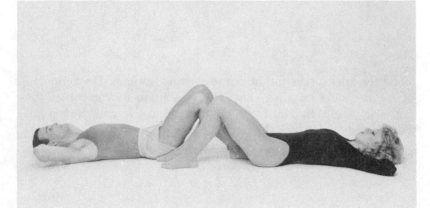

Lie on your backs, with your arms laced under your heads. Locking the right legs as shown, pull your stomachs in tight and hold for 10 counts. Relax and then squeeze your buns tight for another 10 counts.

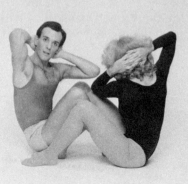

Now sit up and try to touch each other's left elbows. Lie back and immediately come up again to touch right elbows. Challenge each other to sitting up and twisting for a minimum of 8 times.

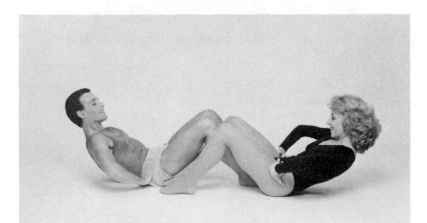

Now place your hands on your hips and sit up 40° off the floor. Hold for 5 counts. Pressing the insides of the right legs together makes it easier and more fun.

CHALLENGE: 10 sit-ups, holding each for 5 counts. No resting in between. Now you can both lie back and curse for a few seconds. Your abdominals will be too shocked to hear you.

This one is great for Buns and Quads. It's good for stomach muscles, too, as it will probably make you laugh a lot.

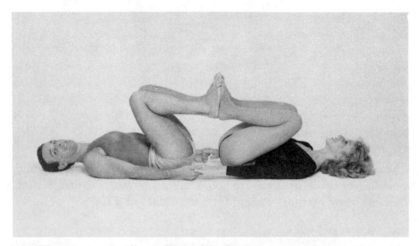

Lie flat on your backs, holding hands. Press your feet against your partner's.

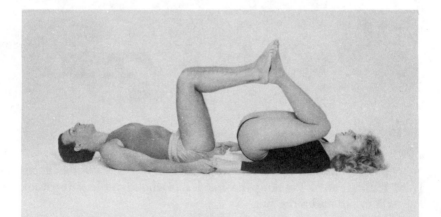

Push partner's feet until her knees touch her chest. She should press back with light resistance.

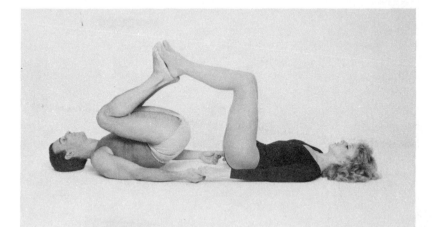

Now it's her turn to do the same to you. Go back and forth at least 10 times each.

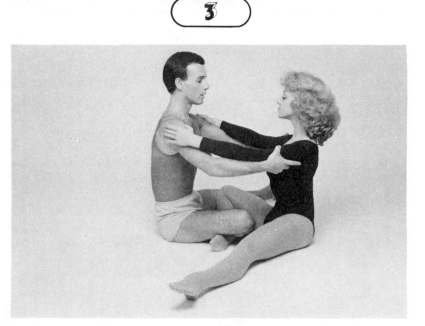

Now we're getting fresh! Lock knees and arms as shown. Try to keep your backs straight. Then, keeping at arm's length, twist your torsos to both sides for 8 counts.

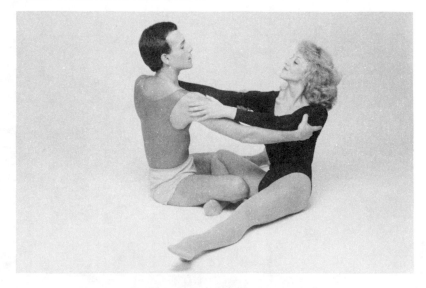

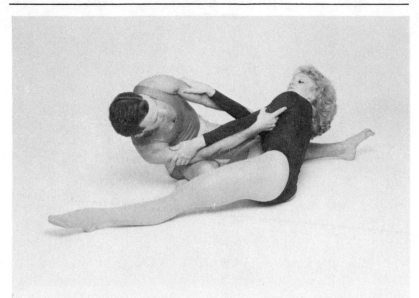

After 8 twists, lean toward each other's extended leg. Sit straight up, then each of you lean toward your own extended leg. Repeat 3 times.

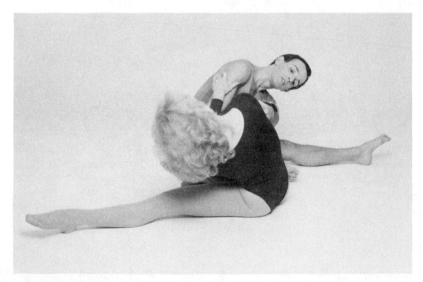

Now lock with the other leg and start all over.

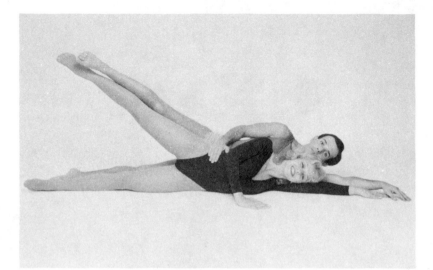

Lie on your sides, back to front. The back partner places his leg on top of the front partner and applies light pressure. The front partner raises her leg toward the ceiling, lifting the back partner's leg. Do a minimum of 16 lifts.

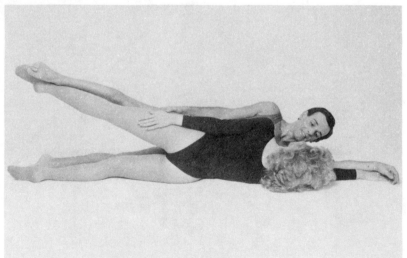

Now turn around and face each other to work the other leg. No kissing allowed—it restricts breathing!

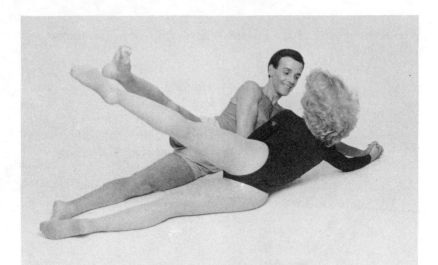

Still facing each other, now hold hands, and while kicking the leg sideways use your arms to push your torsos off the floor. Ester will appreciate it.

Roll over one another—ooops!—and try other side.

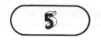

Who is the master of the house? Whoever develops the firmest leg muscles first.

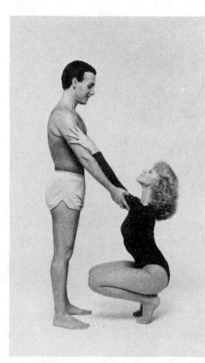

Holding each other at arm's length, let one partner sit while other stands. Then alternate. Do not help each other stand up, please. That's cheating.

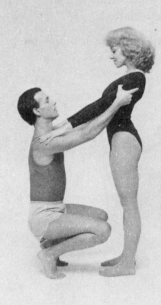

A minimum of 10 for each.

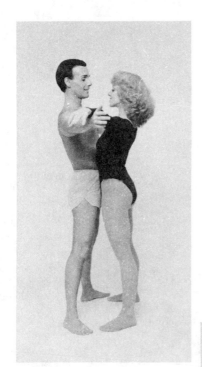

Stand close together with arms extended to the side. No wisecracks please!

From this position, twist torsos from side to side. The more the merrier, but at least 20 times. Be sure to keep your buns and stomach muscles tight.

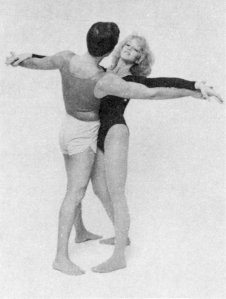

I call this the Fred and Ginger.

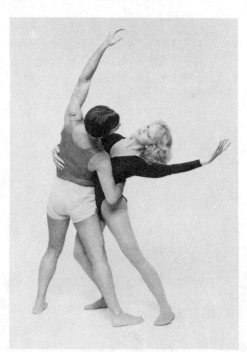

Stand facing each other. Bend opposite knees (if you bend your left, your partner bends her right) and lean away from the bent knees. Support yourselves with an arm wrapped around each other's waist.

Hold onto each other, then quickly switch to the other side. This is a great stretch.

Do a minimum of 8.

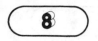

This is the best way to work arms, buns, stomach, and legs without joining a gym (and a sneaky way to tell your partner "No more ice cream").

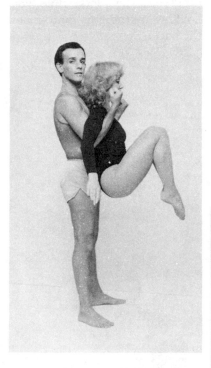

Lock your arms under her arms while she lifts her knees to her chest.

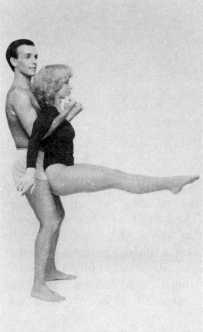

Then bend your knees while she extends legs forward. Hold for 4 counts.

Repeat at least 4 times. (Men, in this age of equality let her take a couple of cracks at it. Ladies, if you can't even get your arms around his stomach, don't even attempt it.)

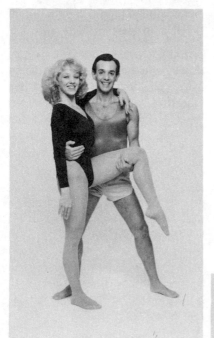

Keep your legs rotated outward from the hip, about 2 or 3 feet apart, and let her put an arm over your shoulders while you hold her by the waist and under the knee.

Bend your knees while she lifts her standing leg straight up. Then stand up while she places her leg on the floor again. Repeat 5 times. Try the other side, too. Remember to keep your stomach tight and back straight. I wouldn't let her try it unless she's unusually strong or you have a hard mattress under you!

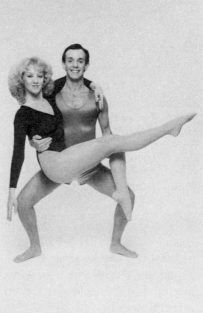

If the difference between your weights is more than 30 pounds, or one of you has either a weak back or Pear Buns, I would skip this one.

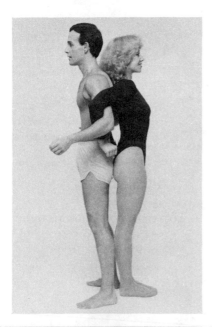

Standing back to back, lock arms.

Bend your knees slightly and lean forward to carry your partner on your back, while she lifts her knees up to her chest.

Ladies, you never know when this one will be handy for either self-defense or "asking" for a favor.

Maximum of 3 times each.

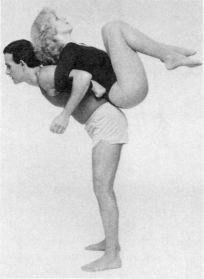

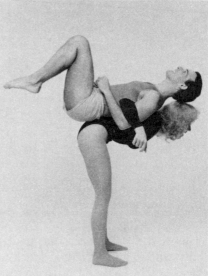

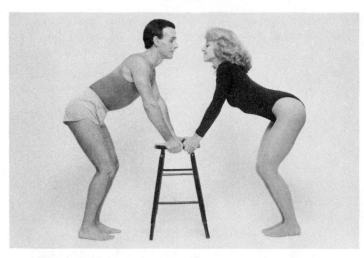

Use a stool or chair and lean on it, keeping your arms straight. Keep your knees bent.

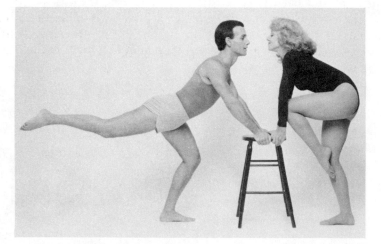

One of you raise your knee forward while the other kicks back, then alternate.

This is the Bunnetics equivalent of the Battle of the Bulge. Stop only when you are out of gas, but never before a minimum of 16 kicks each.

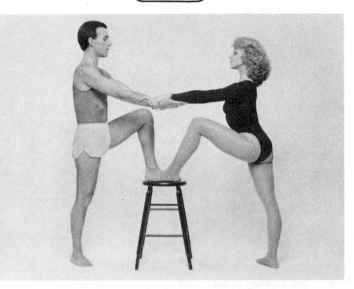

Placing the insides of the feet together (your left and her left, or your right and her right) on the stool, and holding hands, one of you lean your weight forward over your bent knee while the other pulls as far back as possible. The person leaning forward should keep the back straight to avoid bending at the waist. Then reverse the movement.

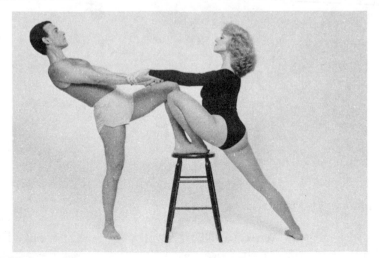

Minimum: 8 forward and 8 back on each side.

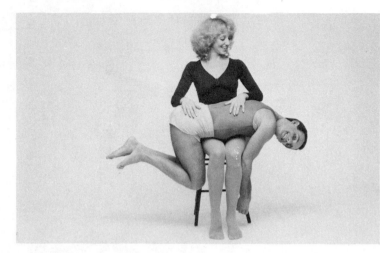

Lie your partner over your thighs and place one hand on his back and the other on his buns to keep him put. Let him stretch out to a horizontal position and have him hold it for 4 counts. Then he should fold down again.

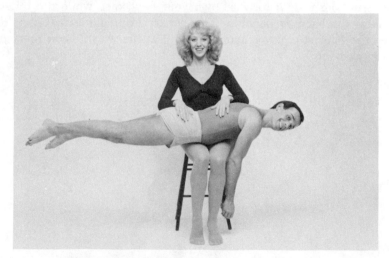

Minimum: 8 horizontal stretches.

Now it's your turn. Wipe that silly grin off your face and make her do at least 8 horizontal stretches.

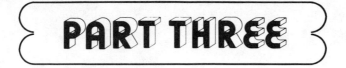

PART THREE

The Unconscious Gulping

While weight loss depends on decreased intake of calories, weight control depends on regulated eating habits and increased physical activity. Losing weight is not that easy, and keeping it off is even harder. Don't let anyone tell you different. Both take more work than just *wanting* to be thin. You actually have to develop an obsession with being skinny. For this reason, weight reduction could drive you into a nervous breakdown unless you make it as easy and as much fun as possible. A trim and healthy body is always attractive, and those who own one waste no time in letting you know it. Show-offs!

So bunners, stand up and turn around. Let your back seat do the driving—straight out of the kitchen!

Big Buns Have Big Eyes

Unquestionably one major reason for our bad eating habits is the gulping down of food with our eyes first. "If it looks yummy, it belongs in the tummy." Wrong! What you see is not what you should always get. Another misused habit is constant snacking. Research studies have shown that Americans make food contact an average of twenty times a day. Snacking is not bad. As a matter of fact, I recommend it as long as you use the right foods for your little-bitty-eating and the total calories from your snacks do not exceed your daily allowance.

It is also a fact that too many people believe that eating well is a sign of prosperity and good living. These folks confuse good eating with large amounts of food on the table, which to them means taking advantage of a fat paycheck. But family customs and ethnic backgrounds are probably the biggest culprits in the formation of bad eating habits. For instance, in most Italian families if you are over thirty and your buns are not large enough to anchor you around the table during never-ending family eat-a-thons, there has to be something wrong with you. The family immediately sets out the cure: tons of pasta and gallons of wine. And who hasn't heard of Jewish mothers? These fabulous ladies bake and matchmake with identical dexterity, influence most of the members of the American Medical Association and the Bar Association, and have time to preach the replacement of penicillin with chicken soup and cigarettes with matzoh balls. Come to think of it, not a bad idea. And although I would love to give examples of all the various groups and their influence on our eating, I must stop with the Latins. (If I don't include them, my mother would certainly never cook for me again.) Somewhere along the line someone told my people that when Ponce de León found the Fountain of Youth (did he?) it was flowing with rice and beans—but for breakfast, lunch, and dinner?

Aside from family customs and financial status, a lot of our eating patterns are part of a habitual chain of reflexes. We have habits that are influenced by various other patterns that affect our gain-loss cycle—work, home life, leisure, depression, happiness, etc. *Any effective change in eating habits must be accompanied by an awareness of the reasons you overeat, the times when you do it, and then a gradual but strong plan that could change both.* It is important to take into consideration the times we eat when we don't plan to, and thus forget we have eaten. This is common with people who have an active social schedule as part of their job, as well as with those with too much free time on their hands.

All of these reasons play a part in our "unconscious gulping" and are the ones to blame for most of the added inches and pounds that increase as you get older and life gradually becomes more sedentary, or bunnentary.

The Disaster Food Diary

There are lots of reasons why people put on weight, and lots of solutions to the problem of overweight. Frankly, I don't really know which is the best solution, but I do know of a way that has worked for me and is recommended by nutritionists. It is a Food Diary.

As a simple and effective aid to record what you eat, and balance and control your weight, the Diary will be your dancer's mirror. It will reflect any disastrous habits and help you to correct them.

When I had to lose weight I devised my own diary from the books I read, and now preach its use to people who come to me with a little too much twirl.

All you need to fill out the Diary are some basic calculations. The figures obtained from them act as the Diary's working guidelines. All of them are approximations, although not far from the actual more exact figures obtained from intricate medical examinations. The things you must learn to find are: ideal weight, basal metabolic rate, daily calorie expenditure, daily calorie deficiency, and daily calorie intake.

IDEAL WEIGHT: The problem with this term seems to be that its word composition, and thus its meaning, is misleading. It implies that a given figure, derived from the heights of people who have lived long and healthy lives, is the ideal target to shoot for by people of identical height and age. These statistics, in the form of charts, are widely used by life insurance companies and physicians alike. But, of course, "ideal weight" depends on various other factors, such as body frame, muscle, and body fat in addition to height, sex, and age. Profession is another factor. A fashion model, a dancer, or a football player's ideal weight can't possibly be the same as that of an average person of their same height. Through my own research I found the following to be the simplest and most general guideline to find your Ideal Weight.

Women: Should weigh 100 pounds for the first 5′ in height, and 5 pounds for every additional inch.

Men: Should weigh 110 pounds for the first 5′ in height, and 5 pounds for every additional inch.

DAILY CALORIE INTAKE: To find these figures you will need a Calorie Count Chart. There are several good ones on the market, the best and most recent of which provide brand names as well. Among these I recommend *Barbara Kraus' Calories and Carbohydrates, Fourth Edition.*

METABOLISM: This is the process by which our body converts the food we eat and the oxygen we breathe into energy and then utilizes it for maintenance and growth. The measure of energy in metabolism is the calorie. Our metabolism rises about an hour after we eat, reaches a maximum about three hours later, and then goes down after the sixth to eighth hour. Different foods cause various levels of metabolic rise. Carbohydrates and fats produce the least and proteins the most. Besides food, muscular activity increases our metabolism more than any other single factor.

BASAL METABOLIC RATE: This is the amount of energy your body burns while at rest. Whether you are counting sheep or Farrah Fawcett's curls, your vital organs must continue to work. Depending on physiological conditions and physical activity, the basal metabolism can account for one half to three quarters of your Daily Energy Output. Basal metabolism also depends on size, age, and sex, with women having a lower one than men of the same age and size. It is estimated that an adult requires 1 calorie per kilogram of weight per hour. Being that a kilogram is equal to 2.2 pounds, a general rule used to find Basal Metabolism Rate is to multiply the Ideal Weight in kilograms by 24, which represents the hours in a day. Hence, the following formula: 1 calorie $\times$ Ideal Weight (in kilograms) $\times$ 24 hours = BMR. It must be noted that in using this formula to restrict caloric intake one must realize that the Ideal Weight already represents less than one's actual weight. Thus, the Basal Metabolic Rate obtained would be considerably lower than the actual one.

DAILY ENERGY OUTPUT: Everything you do in a day, from housework to flying a kite, uses energy. By knowing your BMR plus the average amount of energy burned throughout your active-awake period, you can find your Daily Energy Output (DEO). The amount obtained will vary on a daily basis as you increase physical activity and/or decrease your weight. There are various charts where you can find the amount of energy expenditure of almost every kind of physical activity from running to sex—by the minute or the hour. Based on the fact that BMR accounts for from one half to three quarters of your Daily Energy Output, I have constructed the following groups to help you get a working figure for your Disaster Diary.

Within each group I have written certain descriptions of the jobs they are most likely to represent. Each group has a Level of Vigor, to which percentages are allocated. This is your Daily Activity Quotient and it characterizes the strength or energy you give to your job. Select one and multiply it by your Basal Metabolic Rate. (Example: Your BMR is 1,800. You belong in the Sedentary to Light group, and your Level of Vigor is 40 percent of 1,800. That comes to 720, which you then add to the 1,800 to get a Daily Energy Output of 2,520.) Keep in mind that unless you lead a very methodical life (which good buns will change) you will burn different amounts of energy on different days. This is why you must do your tabulation on a daily basis.

My Days Are:

SEDENTARY TO LIGHT: A day of relaxing or sitting a lot.
Nine-to-five desk or office work.
Bored single or married person who watches three soaps a day.
Level of Vigor: 40%, 42.5%, 50%

MODERATE TO ACTIVE: General housework.
Work requiring moderate manual work.
Standing or walking a lot.
Housewife praying for a maid.
Head of large household wishing to be single.
Level of Vigor: 55%, 57.5%, 60%

VIGOROUS TO STRENUOUS: Lots of physical activity.
A day of participating in sports.
Body-conscious swinging single.
Mayor of a large city.
World's Trade Center window washer.
Level of Vigor: 65%, 70%, 75%

DEFICIT AND SURPLUS: This is simple. If your Daily Calorie Intake exceeds your Daily Energy Output, you have a surplus of calories; if it is under, you have a deficit. Need I say this last one is your goal? Thirty-five hundred calories equals 1 pound of fat. So if you can keep a daily deficit of 500 calories you will lose about 1 pound per week. This balancing is the Diary's main objective.

FAT-OUT WEEKLY SHELTER: Somewhere at the bottom of your Diary keep a running total of your daily deficits. Circle it. At the week's end this shelter acts as a reminder of how you're doing and a projection of your weight loss.

To summarize:

Disaster Food Diary

1. Write down the date and whether it is a work or off day.
2. Glutton Log: Write down everything you have eaten and drunk from morning to retiring. Include the time of the day so you can find out your weakest unconscious gulping periods.
3. Daily Calorie Intake: Add up the values for the day and enter the total.
4. Calculations: Write your "Ideal Weight" and its value in kilograms. Then use the formula to find your BMR and the formula for your DCO.
5. Daily Calorie Output: Enter the figure from No. 4.
6. Deficit (—) Surplus (+): Subtract No. 3 from No. 5. If your Calorie Intake is in excess of your Daily Energy Output, add a plus (+) mark; if it's below, a minus (—).
7. Fill in the Fat-Out Weekly Shelter.

Buy yourself a notebook and make out enough forms for five weeks.

To make it even easier, here are a couple of examples.

Example No. 1:
Your BMR is 1,500 and today you just sat around the house, paid bills, baked cookies, tasted some, watched television, and drank bloody marys. You spent a few hours on the phone while tasting a few more cookies. You weren't just bunnentary, you were a lethargic disgrace! So you take the figure of 40 percent, and I am being generous, and multiply it by 1,500. The result is 600 which you add to the BMR. Your Daily Output is 2,100. But being that you stuffed your stomach to the tune of 3,600 calories, giving you a surplus of 1,500, you will find the next time you sit to pay bills the pen won't fit between your fingers. You sweet fat thing, shame on you!

Example No. 2:
Your BMR is 1,500 and today you played Tarzan. You went to the river and swam all morning, then installed the fireplace in the new tree house, went back to the river and did the laundry on the

rocks, after which you had a couple of rounds of tennis with Jane. You lost, and wildly upset, you went tree swinging with Chita (and I don't mean Rivera). If after a day like this you did not need assistance from your local paramedic tribe, look under Vigorous to Strenuous. Take 75 percent of 1,500 and then add the result to it. It should be 2,625. During this day you lived on a couple of Chita's bananas and some lettuce, not even 220 calories. Your DEO exceeds your caloric Intake by 2,405. A few days like this and the energy burned from your buns could clean the New York City subways.

The Dancer's Skinny Eating

Personally I don't think there are too many professions in which people know as much about food as the dance profession. In New York, dancers spend their lives either trying to find work, or working in a show or dance company. During their quest they go through more struggle, frustration, and expenditure of physical energy than most people realize. All of these contribute to their Skinny Eating Habits.

While there are many types of dancers and dance-related jobs, I must single out the type I am most familiar with: the Broadway dancer. In the past we were called Gypsies because our job was "just to dance" wherever and whenever we had an opportunity. Going from job to job—and often having to travel great distances to pound the boards of the stage—we lived out of a suitcase or a shoulder bag—the Dance Bag. That hasn't changed much. But as past Gypsies escalated the steps of the dance ladder and became director-choreographers, such as Onna White, Agnes de Mille, Herbert Ross, Bob Fosse, Michael Bennett, and others, the Gypsy's job became harder. Because of the experiences and demands of these creative people, as well as the rising costs of mounting a show, today's Gypsy must act and sing in addition to dancing to the same old tunes. And although the name Gypsy remains, it is more an endearment than a classification. And because of the diversity of their trade, some would rather be called artists or entertainers—but none would refuse being called a dancer.

Dancers' eating habits revolve around their work schedule, which is one of constant moving. Remember that to us work doesn't necessarily mean "paid job." The paid job is the easy part. Work consists of the daily things we have to do in order to get a paid job. We take about two, two-hour dance classes a day, varying between ballet, modern dance, jazz dance, and tap dance. Then we have at least two singing and a couple of acting classes a week, plus walking daily all over the city going to auditions, agent interviews, etc. These we manage to do in between our studies and in addition to earning a living through a variety of jobs. All of these physical and psychological efforts are to support our goal—that of being in a hit show! And then when we do get on a stage, it is not rare to find ourselves dancing for five minutes and being used as props for the duration of the show. Fun, isn't it? We wouldn't have it any other way.

Because of our life style, three meals a day are an unheard-of luxury—though I assure you we eat all the time. Why don't we gain weight? Oh, from time to time we do, but as trained artists we know how to camouflage it until we get it off. Of course, to us, gaining weight could mean anything from 6 ounces to 5 pounds. Anything over that could be suicidal.

Our Skinny Eating best friend and food counselor is our Dance Bag. Just as a doctor carries a stethoscope and has a brisk walk, a dancer wouldn't dare step out of the house without a shoulder bag, or Dance Bag. In them we carry enough junk to dress, feed, blow dry, and freshen up the entire New York City corps de ballet. The moment the bag goes on, the feet duck out, head goes up, shoulders go down, and buns tighten to support the bag's weight. But the bag's greatest contribution to weight loss is that *if you can't carry it in the bag—you don't eat it.* This automatically eliminates ice cream, cakes, and pastries unless we are willing to dance in sugar-cured tights.

There is no question in my mind that if you follow the suggestions formulated from the Dancers' Skinny Eating you will learn some slimming habits while losing weight. Although I believe that the only foolproof diet is to just eat less, I feel just as strongly that to do so successfully you must do it gradually.

Don't consider the following suggestions a diet. They aren't. If in order to lose you feel you *must* be on one, there are a lot of good diets around, as well as some scary ones. The Dancers' Skinny Eating suggestions have been formulated from questionnaires filled out by dancers as well as my own observations of the eating habits of my fellow Gypsies. When you lose the weight, remember that thousands of dancers helped you. A trip to New York and seeing a couple of Broadway shows will be more than adequate thanks.

THE MORNING RUSH: I don't think I know anyone who (except on an occasional Sunday morning) sets up a breakfast table and decorates it with the normal egg-bacon-toast-hash browns-juice-milk-coffee combination. But breakfast is an important part of a dancer's day because lunch, as most people know it, is practically unknown. A high-protein meal is the best way to get the energy necessary to propel us through the day, and shakes are favored because they're quick to make and consume. The use of a Protein Powder is featured in all of these breakfast suggestions because of its energy-sustaining value. For calorie counting ease, the shakes are grouped in combinations where the ingredients have about the same caloric value.

Breakfast #1

	CAL.	PROT.	FAT	CAR.
2 tbs. Protein Powder with	110	26	0	1
4 oz. cut up papaya, or	35	1	0	9
4 oz. cut up peaches, or	35	1	0	20
4 oz. fresh strawberries, and	25	1	1	6
8 oz. no-fat or skim milk, or	90	10	2	14
6 ice cubes	0	0	0	0
Average Value:	231	37	2	25

Breakfast #2

2 tbs. Protein Powder with	110	26	0	1
8 oz. orange juice, or	100	1	0	23
8 oz. grapefruit juice, or	100	1	0	23
8 oz. carrot juice, or	90	1	0	20
8 oz. pineapple juice, or	120	0	0	32
8 oz. apple juice, or	120	0	0	32
8 oz. papaya juice	75	1	0	14
6 ice cubes	0	0	0	0
Average Value: (excluding carrot and papaya)	220	27	0	25

Breakfast #3

	CAL.	PROT.	FAT	CAR.
2 tbs. Protein Powder with	110	26	0	1
1 raw egg	80	6	6	0
6 oz. vegetable or tomato juice	35	1	0	8
6 ice cubes	0	0	0	0
Average Value:	225	33	6	9

Breakfast #4 (Hi-Vitality)

	CAL.	PROT.	FAT	CAR.
2 tbs. Protein Powder with	110	26	0	1
8 oz. plain yogurt (no-fat or from skim milk)	110	11	7	14
2 tbs. Wheat Germ, with	110	9	3	13
4 oz. no-fat or skim milk	45	5	1	7
6 ice cubes	0	0	0	0
Average Value:	375	51	11	35

As you can see, Breakfasts 1, 2, and 3 have about the same caloric value, although different nutrient values. If in the morning you must have your coffee and a piece of toast, then you must add 100 calories for each slice, and an additional 50 calories if you butter it. Needless to say, sugar is out of the question. A sugar substitute has a couple of calories, and 1 tbs. of honey has 65 calories and 17 carbohydrates. I, for one, can't do without my coffee and my piece of toast and am addicted to honey.

Breakfast #4 is an extra-high-protein one which I recommend to those who have real determination and can wait until the end of the day to eat, or whose lunch or midday snacks are minimal. Whichever breakfast you choose, remember that you eat it *after* your Buns exercises.

THE MIDDAY BLUES: If you have a high-protein breakfast, there's no real reason why you should have too many hunger pains during the day. But when you must, you must. Keep in mind that it is during the day that the Unconscious Gulping keeps knocking at your stomach's door, and if you are the type that sends for every TV offer or can't keep your door closed to try-now-pay-later salesmen, you are a candidate for the Moby Dick tank.

The number of things you can eat to satisfy your mental hunger is tremendous, as you will see from the list of snacks most liked by dancers. Whether we are taking class or rehearsing a show, it is impossible to dance with a feeling of fullness, so in between classes or on hourly breaks we munch away like mad. If you can keep your munching under 150 calories, you will be doing well, but even 200 calories won't kill you.

From the Dance Bag

	Calories	Protein	Fat	Carbohydrate
1 apple	70	0	0	18
1 banana	85	1	0	23
1 carrot	20	1	0	14
1 celery stalk	5	0	0	2
1 bunch grapes (cup)	65	1	1	15
1 peach	35	1	0	10
1 orange	60	2	0	16
1 tangerine	40	1	1	10
1 lemon	20	1	0	6
1 dill pickle	15	1	0	3
1 cup fresh cherries	80	1	0	6
1 plum	25	0	0	7
½ cantaloupe	60	1	0	14
Nuts & Dried Seeds				
Almonds (1 oz.)	105	3	9	4
Cashews (1 oz.)	95	3	8	5
Peanuts (1 oz.)	105	5	9	3
Sesame Seeds (1 oz.)	110	5	4	6

Although many of us do practically live out of our bags, at least until we get home, I don't want you to think that our eating totally depends on it. Lunch time in the theater district is fun time all through the week, except on Wednesday and Saturday, when matinee goers invade the city. On the other days the area is a melting pot of everyone in show business, from stage hands to box office managers. At this time more lettuce and vegetables are consumed than in all the rabbit farms in the country. Chef's salad (about 400 calories per 4 oz. serving) seems the winner, but yogurt with fruit salad (usually around 250 calories) with all kinds of healthful toppings (more calories) runs a close second. Of course, there are the all-time favorites like tuna salad in a large tomato (225 calories), with a boiled egg and melba toast thrown in for decoration (another 95 calories), and the beef patty and cottage cheese (440 calories). Then there are the very religious dancers who confess to the waiter, "Just tea with lemon," and then whisper, "Pecan pie à la mode" (penance: 650 calories plus 10 Hail Marys). As a note I must add that it is primarily the "presently in a show" theater people whom you will find at places like Ted Hook's Backstage, where "Who made the salad?" is often changed to "What celebrity is eating it?" When you are not working or your show has closed, it's back to plastic containers in your Dance Bag. But the combination of foods remains pretty much the same.

THE NIGHT OWL: Dinner time is definitely the Gypsy's favorite time. It would take a volume just to describe the variety of sumptuous dishes I have consumed at many of my friends' homes. (I might just write them down for you sometime.) What dancers miss during the day they make up for at night. Vegetarianism is very common among theater people, and their dinners almost always end with fruits, nuts, and often cheese. I would dare say that cheeses of all kinds are favored by dancers not only at dinner, but as snacks during the day. Meats are rare, due to the prevalence of vegetarianism as much as cost. Dancers are fish and chicken eaters, and desserts are usually foregone for wine, white wine being without question the dancer's favorite. All in all, we tend to eat protein-rich foods along with good carbohydrates from vegetables, and needed fat from dairy products. The Food and Drug Administration office should be proud of us!

As a closing note, I would like to give you these Dancers' Skinny Eating tips.

1. Eat a good protein breakfast. Try the protein shakes for a quick morning picker-upper.

2. Find out what your "ideal weight" is and try to maintain it.

3. Avoid eating too much fat. Stick to lean meats, fish, and chicken.

4. Do away with empty carbohydrates. Never say, "Sugar Please."

5. Avoid too much salt.

6. If you drink, do it in moderation. Calories from alcohol go straight to your buns.

7. Snacking is good when it is done with fruits and salads.

8. Stay away from drinking sweetened carbonated refreshments. Water is the winner among dancers.

9. Eat slowly and enjoy it more by chewing well.

10. Discover the greatness of yogurt for a slimming and nourishing meal.

11. When you eat alone, you tend to eat more and much faster. A good book, a crossword puzzle, or writing that overdue letter are great meal companions.

12. Eating in bed or just before going to bed is a definite fat gainer. Sweets and clean sheets make ton-like buns.

13. Try to plan your at-home meals well before time—especially those following holidays and weekends. When you must pig-out, check your deficit calorie reservoir in your Fat-Out Shelter.

14. Eat at regular intervals and avoid fasting or skipping meals. Keep your metabolism working for you all day.

15. Use the Bunnetics Disaster Food Diary.

16. Follow the Bunnetics Exercise Plan.

17. Don't leave for tomorrow the buns you could start today; after all, Bunnetics is behind you all the way.

—BUNALE—